Table of Contents

The Med Diet Score

You've probably heard the term "Mediterranean Diet" mentioned in the media, and if you're like most people, the phrase probably makes you think it means eating Greek food, like hummus, Greek salad, and olive oil. Even physicians have been known to say, "Sure, Mediterranean Diet. Olive oil, garlic, and fish."

While all of those foods can be considered part of the Mediterranean Diet, it's as close to a complete picture of the Mediterranean diet as saying that the American diet is burgers and apple pie. It's much more accurate, really, to call it a "Mediterranean-**style** diet," because it's more about a **pattern** of eating than it's about eating specific foods.

Just What is The Mediterranean Diet?

The sheer volume of available nutrition information is a real challenge for Americans wanting to know just how to eat well and still eat healthy. There have been so many different messages in the last 30 years, with some of that misinformation coming from fad diets, which are generally based on faulty science at best and much more often based on myth and pseudoscience. The confusion also comes from the fact that nutrition science has been evolving in the last few years. Consequently, messages founded in good quality science do change over time as we learn more, and thus recommendations can change. Between this and silly fad diets it can be hard to know what to believe.

That's the bad news.

The good news is that there has been a tremendous amount of excellent research about diet and nutrition published in the last decade. We now have a great understanding of what works from studies of Mediterranean style diet. This diet is higher in fruits and nuts, vegetables, legumes (beans and peas), and whole grains and cereals. Followers of a Mediterranean-style diet consume less red meats and poultry as their main animal protein and eat more fish along with some dairy - although much of the dairy is in the form of cultured products like cheeses and yogurt. The lower intake of poultry and red meats is coupled with a moderate consumption of alcohol. For the most part the alcohol consumed is wine, and that is most often with meals.

The main source of fat used is olive oil and there is less use of highly saturated fats like butter and lard - but not none..

The best way for you to think about this is to focus on these ingredients and not specific Mediterranean recipes. These ingredients have formed the basis for Health meets Food recipes, and the diet, for the most part, adds up to fewer calories and better quality foods. That is, in essence, how to think of the MedDiet Score diet. Using the principles of Mediterranean diet, applying them to the American kitchen, and translating recipes that you know and love into delicious, health-giving meals that will sustain you in both body and soul.

Prior to the turn of the 20th century there had been a number of studies to show just how healthy the Mediterranean Diet was, and in 2003 Antonia Trichopoulou and colleagues reported on a large study that examined over 22,000 healthy adults in Greece and found that those who more closely followed a Mediterranean style diet had a significant reduction in their risk of death due to heart disease and cancer. (1)

While there had been other studies, this was an exhaustive look with the researchers following participants over time. Dr. Trichopoulou and her colleagues analyzed the diets of those in the study for a year prior to the beginning of data collection. They then looked at nine dietary components of a Mediterranean-style Diet: vegetables, legumes, fruits and nuts, whole grains, fish, olive oil (good fats), dairy products (mostly cheese and yogurt), lean meats (including red meat), and alcohol. A value was assigned of either 1 or 0 for each dietary category. If a participant was found to have eaten a diet more favorably in each of the nine dietary components they received a point in each of those categories. The maximum score for a perfect Mediterranean diet would be 9, and a score of 0 would indicate a more Western diet pattern. The also issued a lifestyle questionnaire that recorded physical activity.

The results were pretty amazing. Quite simply? Those who had better scores lived longer.

The best part is that small changes have a big effect. A two-point increase in one's Mediterranean Diet Score - say, from a 5 to a 7 - meant a 25% reduction in death from all causes. This would mean that by making fairly small changes in your diet - say, by simply eating more vegetables and legumes - you could markedly improve your health and live longer.

1. Trichopoulou A, Bamia C, Trichopoulos D. Adherence to a Mediterranean diet and survival in a Greek population. *N Engl J Med.* 2003;348(26):2599-2608. doi:10.1056/NEJMoa025039

Mediterranean Diet and Your Quality of Life

We know that following a Mediterranean style diet can help prevent a number of chronic diseases and conditions, from improving insulin levels and cholesterol scores to preventing heart attack and stroke. But health is more than just lack of disease - it's also about quality of life.

It might sound pretty hard to quantify one's quality of life, but researchers at the RAND Corporation have taken a stab at it by developing what is known as the SF-36, or Short Form Health Survey (36 being the number of questions). The survey is divided into several sections, with sample questions as follows:

- Do you feel full of pep?"
- "Does your health limit you in... lifting or carrying groceries?"
- "How much bodily pain have you had during the past 4 weeks?"
- "In general, would you say your health is...."
- "Have you felt so down in the dumps that nothing could cheer you up?"

These are designed to measure both physical as well as mental well-being.

Researchers in Spain noted that the Mediterranean Diet had a significant impact on physical health. Was it also related to an improved quality of life? They made use of data gathered during a long-term study of university graduates in Navarra, Spain.(1) Over 11,000 men and women participated in responding to detailed food questionnaires as well as taking the SF-36. After four years of followup the researchers assigned each participant a Mediterranean Diet score of 0-9, with 9 being high adherence and 0 being a more Western-style diet. They then correlated the participants' Mediterranean Diet scores with their scores on the SF-36.

Unsurprisingly, they found that those with a higher Mediterranean Diet score indicated a higher physical quality of life. They also reported a better emotional quality of life, although the association was not as strong.

What's interesting is what they discovered when the researchers looked at those whose adherence to the Mediterranean style diet changed over the four years of the study. Increasing one's Mediterranean Diet score by as little as one point meant a fairly significant increase in both their physical and emotional quality of life. The exact amount is hard to quantify - these are very subjective states, after all - but the increase in scores was as little as 10% and as much as 50%.

This study design is considered retrospective, meaning that we look back over time. What about quality of life when the study is designed as an interventional trial? Can a change in diet actually affect your mood? A recent study (2) suggests that a Mediterranean Diet may help improve more than just your body's health - it may help improve your mood.

Researchers in Australia recruited 25 women between the ages of 19 and 30 to participate in a 10-day study. At the start of the study all of the participants responded to two questionnaires to assess their mood: first, a standardized questionnaire designed to measure an individual's mood in six dimensions: Depression, Anxiety, Anger, Vigor, Fatigue, and Confusion. A second questionnaire assessed three mood factors: Alert, Calm, and Content. A standardized mental performance assessment tested changes in cognition; measuring attention, working memory, long term memory, and executive function.

Half of the women were assigned to a Diet Change group, while the other half were asked to continue their normal diet for the succeeding ten days. The Diet Change group received an eating plan, which specified the foods they should eat (and which they should avoid eating) for the ten days of the study. These women were asked to increase the amount of fruit, nuts, vegetables, fatty fish and whole grain cereals, while avoiding red meat, refined sugar and flour, pre-packaged or processed foods, all caffeinated products and soft drinks (note the similarity to Mediterranean diet). The number of calories they were to eat was not controlled and the women in both groups kept a food diary for the ten days of the study.

After ten days the two mood questionnaires and the cognitive tests were administered again and the results compared to the earlier outcomes.

Those women in the Diet Change group reported greater feelings of Vigor, while Alertness increased in the Diet Change group and actually decreased in the Usual Diet group. Most interestingly, those in the Usual Diet group reported lower feelings of Contentedness at the end of the study, while those who followed a Mediterranean Diet reported higher feelings of Contentedness.

On the other hand, those in the Usual Diet group performed two of the cognitive tasks more quickly at the end of the study than at the start, while those in the Diet Change group did not improve their scores. In only one cognitive test did the Diet Change group improve while the Usual Diet group did not.

Certainly this is a very small study and its design could be improved by providing all meals to all of the participants rather than allowing them to choose their own foods. But its results with regard to mood are intriguing: healthier may well mean happier.

1. European Journal of Clinical Nutrition 66, 360 (2012). doi:10.1038/ejcn.2011.146
2. Mcmillan L, Owen L, Kras M, Scholey A. Behavioural effects of a 10-day Mediterranean diet. Results from a pilot study evaluating mood and cognitive performance. Appetite. 2011;56(1):143-147. doi:10.1016/j.appet.2010.11.149.

Your Mediterranean Diet Score

What about those 9 components of the Mediterranean diet? How has this been used in research and what does it mean for you? What makes up the Mediterranean diet score?

That study of over 22,000 Greeks mentioned above determined a threshold amount for each component of the Mediterranean Diet. The following list details those thresholds and you can calculate your own diet score based on these amounts.

It is pretty simple. The scores have been adjusted for a 1,500 calorie per day diet for women and 1,800 calories for men. For instance, if you are a woman and consume more than 9 ounces of veggies by weight per day, on average over a week, you score one point. Eat less than that on average and you get zero. The best overall score is a 9 and the worst a zero.

Work through these 9 sections and see how you score. Keep track of your food intake for a week and score yourself on the average over the week. Even better, you'll find that keeping a simple food diary can help you identify places where you can improve your score.

1. If you are female, do you eat more than 9 ounces of vegetables per day (11 ounces for men)?
> 4 ounces is about two medium carrots
> 4 ounces is about 8 medium spears of asparagus
> 4 ounces is about 1 cup sliced yellow squash or zucchini
> 4 ounces is about one 3 inch beet
> 4 ounces is about 1 1/4 cups chopped broccoli

Score:
> 1 point for more than 9 ounces female / 11 ounces male
>
> 0 points for less than 9 ounces female / 11 ounces male

2. Do you eat more than 1 3/4 ounces of legumes per day (2 ounces for men)?
> 1 3/4 ounces is about 1/4 cup canned chick peas
> 1 3/4 ounces is about 3 tablespoons peanut butter
> 1 3/4 ounces is about 1/4 cup raw lentils
> 1 3/4 ounces is about 1/3 cup canned kidney beans
> 1 3/4 ounces is about 1/3 cup roasted soybeans
> 2 ounces is about 2/3 cup frozen peas

Score:
> 1 point for more than 1 3/4 ounces female / 2 ounces male

3. Do you eat more than 8 ounces of fruits or nuts per day (9 ounces for men)?
> 8 ounces is 1 large apple
> 8 ounces is 2 medium bananas

Score:
> 1 point for more than 8 ounces female / 9 ounces male
> 0 points for less than 8 ounces female / 9 ounces male

4. Do you eat more than 9 ounces of cereals or grains per day (10 1/2 ounces for men)?
> 2 ounces is about 1 cup bite size shredded wheat
> One slice of whole wheat bread is 1 ounce
> 1/4 cup of uncooked brown rice is about 2 ounces
> 1/2 cup dry whole wheat pasta is about 2 ounces
> 1/3 cup uncooked quinoa is about 2 ounces

Score:
> 1 point for more than 9 ounces female / 10 1/2 ounces male
> 0 points for less than 9 ounces female / 10 1/2 ounces male

5. Do you eat more than 3/4 ounces of fish per day (1 ounces for men)?
This is not very much, but the research looked at averages: that's why it seems to be so little. This really means about two or more 4 ounce servings per week.

Score:
> 1 point for more than 3/4 ounces female / 1 ounce per day male
> 0 point for less than 3/4 ounces female / 1 ounce per day male

6. The ratio of the type of fat you consume is important. Do you eat more healthy oils? The optimal ratio is 1.6 portions of healthy fat to 1 portion of less healthy.

Examples of healthy fats:
> Olive oil
> Canola oil
> Grapeseed oil
> Peanut oil
> Soybean oil

Examples of less healthy fats:
> Hydrogenated vegetable oil
> Stick or hard margarines
> Butter
> Lard
> Vegetable shortening

Score:
1 point for greater than the optimum ratio of greater than 1.6 to 1 for healthy fats:less healthy fats.
0 point for less than the optimum ratio of greater than 1.6 to 1 for healthy fats:less healthy fats.

7. Do you eat less than 7 ounces of dairy per day (7 1/4 ounces for men)?
7 ounces is by weight and is about a cup of yogurt or a glass of milk

Score:
> 1 point for less than 7 ounces female / 7 1/4 ounces male
> 0 point for more than 7 ounces female / 7 1/4 ounces male

8. Do you eat less than 3 1/4 ounces of meat per day (4 ounces for men)?
Most people think that a serving of meat is much larger than it should be. Four ounces of beef, chicken, pork or lamb is about the size of a deck of cards.

Score:
> 1 point for less than 3 1/4 ounces female / 4 ounces male
> 0 points for more than 3 1/4 ounces female / 4 ounces male

9. Do you drink between 5 and 25 grams of alcohol per day (10 and 50 grams for men)?
25 grams is the equivalent of about one drink:
> One twelve ounce beer
> One 5 ounce glass of wine
> One 1 ounce shot of spirits

Score:
> 1 point for between 5 and 25 grams female / 10 and 50 grams male
> 0 point for less than 5 grams female / 10 grams male

Subtract 1 point for more than 25 grams female / 50 grams male

Conclusion and Score

There is no passing or failing grade for this test. The higher your score the better. A perfect Mediterranean style diet would be a score of 9 and if you're living off snack food and soda, it is likely your score will be closer to zero.

The impact of improving your score can be dramatic. One of the largest Mediterranean diet studies showed that a two point increase in your score, from 5 to 7, translates to a 25% reduction in the risk of death from heart disease or cancer.

Moderation is the Key

Eating healthier is not just quality but also moderation. This doesn't always mean what you think: I believe that it means most of the time you are eating great food and occasionally splurging, but this also means finding that middle ground between the extremes of highly restrictive, deprivation diets and eating at Applebee's every day.

A good example of that middle ground was demonstrated by researchers at Loma Linda University.(1) Their large-scale, long-term study includes over 77,000 Seventh Day Adventists, who are directed by their faith to follow a diet that avoids meat and includes "legumes, whole grains, nuts, fruits, and vegetables" (Adventist.org: www.adventist.org/vitality/health/). Adventists participating in the study were recruited from all 50 states in the U.S. as well as all of the Canadian provinces and include adults 25 and older. The baseline questionnaire for all participants included an extensive food frequency questionnaire that allowed the researchers to classify the participants into 5 different dietary patterns. The end point, or measure of health, for this particular analysis was the likelihood of developing colorectal cancers in the five groups analyzed:

Vegan (defined as consuming eggs, dairy, fish, or other meats less than once per month);
Lacto-Ovo Vegetarian (defined as consuming eggs or dairy at least once per month and consuming fish or meats less than once per month)
Pescetarian (consuming fish at least once per month but eating all other meats less than once per month)
Semivegetarians (ate animal proteins less than once per week);
Nonvegetarians (ate animal proteins 1 time per week or more).

After an average of 7 years of follow-up, the researchers could compare the dietary patterns of those who developed colorectal cancers with those who did not. You might expect that vegans would be the least likely to develop colorectal cancers, given its avoidance of animal protein and high levels of fruits and veg-etables along with legumes and whole grains. Not so!

After taking into account age, Body Mass Index (BMI), family history of colorectal cancer or peptic ulcer, Vitamin D or calcium supplement intake, and total fiber consumption, among other variables, those who saw the lowest risk of colorectal cancers were the pescetarians with a 42% reduction in risk. Vegans, however, reduced their risk by only 14%, while lacto-ovo vegetarians lowered their risk by 17%.

Once again, prospective studies like these do not necessarily prove a causal link, but it's hard to escape the conclusion that the only difference between two of the dietary patterns - one eating fish, the other not - must have significant impact. What exactly that might be (omega-3 or omega-6 acids? iodine content? something else?) is still up for some debate.

In the end, this means that a more restrictive diet is not necessarily better for you.

There has been similar research showing that those who consume a moderate amount of alcohol, mostly with meals, are less likely to develop diabetes or heart disease than those who do not consume alcohol, (2).while those whose intake is excessive (4 or more drinks per day for women, or 4 1/2 drinks per day for men) are almost twice as likely to develop diabetes. One theory is that it's the antioxidants in wine that confer the protective effects, although we also know that all types of alcohol (wine, beer, or liquor) help reduce the markers of inflammation that are associated with chronic conditions like diabetes, heart disease, and cancer.

That said, the risk of developing gastro-esophageal (esophagus and stomach) cancers is slightly higher among those who drink. A study in the *American Journal of Clinical Nutrition* looks at alcohol use and survival in those diagnosed with colorectal cancers (3).

The authors used information gathered through an ongoing study in Germany. Over 3,000 men and women who had recently been diagnosed for the first time with colorectal cancer (CRC) responded to demographic, medical, and lifestyle history questionnaires that included estimates of the participant's alcohol intake, both in the past (at ages 20, 30, 40, etc.) and within the year just prior to their diagnosis.

For the following 5 years, on average, the authors were updated by the patients' physicians regarding treatment and recurrence, and causes of death for those patients who died during those five years were collected from their local public health departments. The participants' alcohol intake was defined as "abstainers" (those who did not drink at all), "light drinkers" (up to 1 drink per day for women and up to 2 for men), "moderate drinkers" (between 1 and 2 drinks per day for women, 2-4 for men), and "heavy drinkers" (more than 2 drinks per day for women, more than 4 drinks per day for men).

The authors found that compared to light drinkers, those who abstained from drinking any alcohol over their whole lives had lower rates of overall five-year survival (meaning they did not die of any cause) and much lower rates of CRC-specific survival (dying from colorectal cancer specifically).

On the other hand, compared to light drinkers, heavy drinkers also had lower rates of overall survival and were far less likely to survive disease-free for the five years of follow-up. This tendency for abstainers and heavier drinkers to fare less well than those who were light or moderate drinkers held true across the various outcomes the authors considered, from risk of recurrence to risk of death from CRC.

This study does mirror the other positive effects of moderate alcohol intake and should be considered all the more reason to keep both your drinking and food consumption moderate.

1. Orlich MJ, Singh PN, Sabaté J, et al. Vegetarian Dietary Patterns and the Risk of Colorectal Cancers. *JAMA Intern Med.* 2015;175(5):767-10
2. Nettleton. Dietary Flavonoids and Flavonoid-Rich Foods Are Not Associated with Risk of Type 2 Diabetes in Postmenopausal Women1. *J Nutr.* November 2006:7.
3. Walter V, Jansen L, Ulrich A, et al. Alcohol consumption and survival of colorectal cancer patients: a population-based study from Germany. *Am J Clin Nutr.* 2016;103(6):1497-1506. doi:10.3945/ajcn.115.127092

Questions For You...

Answer the following questions for yourself:

1. What are you doing tomorrow at 2:00 pm?
2. How about next Tuesday at 9:00 am?
3. And the day after that at noon?

Invariably people know the answers to these sorts of questions. Sometimes they know off the top of their heads, other times it takes a bit of thought, and some people will pull out their smart phones and check their calendar.

Now answer this question:

4. What are you having for lunch today?

Most of us believe that we don't have a lot of time to cook these days. However, cooking three to four times a week is doable. It is important to remember that making great food for yourself and your family does take some commitment of time and that investment will pay off.

The question for you is "what are you having for dinner tonight?" When you can answer that the vast majority of the time you will see a major improvement in your health. The second step is to make sure that you are making the right choices for breakfast, lunch, dinner, snacks, and beverages.

Cooking at Home is Cheaper and Better for You

The Seattle Obesity Study surveyed 437 adult men and women who did the bulk of the food shopping in their household (1). Not only were they asked to estimate how often, on average, they and members of their family ate outside the home, they were also asked how much they spent on food (including both at home and away from home). Further, they responded to a dietary questionnaire regarding their diet as a whole that the authors could then score against the USDA's Healthy Eating Index (HEI 2010), which measures how well one's diet adheres to the Dietary Guidelines for Americans. Scored from 0 to 100, a higher score means a greater adherence.

In analyzing the data, the authors took into account not only age, gender, race/ethnicity, marital status, and number of people in the household, but also income, education, and employment status (employed versus unemployed).

Somewhat unsurprisingly, those who were unmarried, lived alone, or did not have children ate out most often. About half of all respondents reported eating at home "frequently" (6 or more times per week), with one third cooking 4-5 times per week. (It's encouraging to see that only 15% of the sample said they cooked 3 or fewer times per week - that's a lot of eating out.) Those who were married, had more people in the household (adult or child), had at least one child in the household, or were unemployed were more likely to eat at home more often.

Also unsurprisingly: eating at home more often meant a better HEI 2010 score, with those who ate at home frequently having an average score 7 points higher than those who ate at home rarely. The authors looked at the various components of the HEI score and found that those who ate at home consumed fewer total calories, fewer empty calories, and less sodium than those who ate out, with the amount of total protein in the diet being the only component that was about the same between eating at home or away from home.

Finally, those who cooked at home spent most of their total food expenditures on foods they would eat at home: only 23% of their total food budget was spent on food eaten away from home. By contrast, those who ate out the most didn't spend their money in the same proportion of home versus away: 53% of their food money was spent at home, while 47% was spent away from home. Overall, those who ate at home the most spent 17% less on their food bills each month than those who ate out the most.

1. Tiwari A, Aggarwal A, Tang W, Drewnowski A. Cooking at Home_ A Strategy to Comply With U.S. Dietary Guidelines at No Extra Cost. *AMEPRE*. 2017;52(5):616-624. doi:10.1016/j.amepre.2017.01.017.

Planning is Everything

There are a lot of diets out there. The research says that most all of them are successful - at least when the measure of success is weight loss. The issue is that with most of the plans people stop using them mostly because they are so restrictive — cut out carbs, don't eat wheat, liquids only for breakfast and lunch. At the same time they don't really teach you anything about how to eat.

The one thing that they all have in common is that they are a plan. It is the plan that is the key to their short term success, but few offer any way forward with long term sustainability. They don't teach you how to make your own plans or how to implement them.

Most of my patients don't know what they're going to have for lunch, and too often that means choosing their lunch by looking at a menu and choosing the first thing that looks good. And that, as you probably know, is unlikely to be the healthiest choice you could be making.

Yet time and again research has shown us that planning is everything.

For example, researchers at the Center for Urban Health Policy partnered with the Health and Wellness department of Einstein Healthcare Network in Pennsylvania to find ways to help people make healthier choices at lunchtime (1). They recruited participants for a study from the staff at a large urban hospital in Philadelphia that had an employee cafeteria where many of the staff were accustomed to having their lunch. The 26 participants were all overweight or obese, willing to eat at least three times per week in the hospital cafeteria, and also willing to allow the researchers to collect data about their lunch purchases from the cafeteria.

The researchers theorized that ordering one's lunch in advance - at least 45 minutes before picking it up from the cafeteria - might lead to eating fewer calories at lunch. They worked with the cafeteria food provider, Aramark, to create an online ordering tool, complete with nutrition information for each food (which was not available at the physical cafeteria) that would allow participants to choose their lunch each day from the current day's offerings. The single requirement was that the order must be placed at least 45 minutes in advance of pickup.

After an initial four to eight weeks of monitoring the participants' usual purchases at the cafeteria, the researchers provided the participants with mindful eating training, which includes strategies to help avoid emotional eating and being more present and less distracted (by television or other media, for example) while actually eating. For the following four weeks the participants were provided with discount coupons to encourage their use of the system, then for an additional four weeks they were encouraged to continue using the system without the coupons.

After the full 8 weeks, the researchers could compare the participants' usual average caloric intake with the selections they made using the advance ordering tool. They found that on average, when the participants were using coupons, they ordered about 70 fewer calories than they usually would. When they were NOT using coupons, however, they reduced their average number of lunch calories by about 115 calories. Similarly, they reduced their fat intake by as much as 5 grams of fat.

Note that the participants were not given instruction in nutrition and that the mindfulness training has nothing to do with being mindful of caloric intake. Simply being able to make their lunch choices in advance of lunch time led the participants to choose foods with fewer calories and less fat than they would otherwise.

It may interest you to know that the food you keep at home provides 72%, by weight, of all the food that you eat. This is assuming that you do not prepare most meals at home, however. If you do make most of your meals at home (breakfast and dinner made at home and taking your lunch with you to work or school), then 93% of the food you eat comes from what is kept in your home.

So what? Of course your food comes from what you have at home. Researchers at Rutgers University wondered if there was a difference in what foods were actually in the home between those families with overweight members and those families who were all of normal weight (2). One hundred mothers with at least one child 12 years of age or younger were recruited to participate in the study. These women were all primarily responsible for all meal planning, grocery shopping, and meal preparation, and were either married or living with a domestic partner. In addition, the family unit ate dinner at home at least three times per week.

To assess the quality of food kept in the home, the investigators conducted an inventory of the food in each participant's home. Yes, they literally went into the home and counted every food item in the house, with the exception of such items as condiments and seasonings, bulk items like flour and sugar, baby foods, pet foods, alcoholic beverages and leftovers. The specific item and its amount by weight was recorded for each food, then the investigators computed the total number of calories, protein, fat, saturated fat and so forth present for all foods in the house and divided that total by the recommended daily allowance (for an adult) of each nutrient. This yielded the number of days' worth of the nutrient that was present in each household. The researchers then had a standardized unit of the different nutrients in food so that each household could be fairly compared with others.

Each family member had his or her Body Mass Index calculated by the researchers, who then were able to compare the foods from households with overweight or obese parents (either mother, partner or both) with the foods from households of normal-weight parents.

All of the homes tended to keep the same amounts of nutrients on hand, but the differences were in what forms of foods those nutrients were in. For example, those homes with overweight parents tended to have their carbohydrates in the form of frozen potatoes (like tater tots or french fries) or frozen vegetables with an included sauce (like broccoli with cheese sauce or Brussels sprouts with butter sauce). Fresh and frozen meats also supplied more of the protein, total fat, and saturated fats than in normal-weight households.

It's a saying among nutrition researchers that "people eat **food**, not nutrients." The take-home message here is about the choices the households had made about the type of food brought into the home. Instead of processed potatoes and vegetables, cook them fresh. Choose leaner meats and avoid processed meats so that you get less fat with your animal protein. Choose better foods to have in the house and you'll be healthier (and likely weigh less).

You've probably noticed that it's not a good idea to go grocery shopping when you're hungry. It's all too easy to end up buying a whole bunch of things you didn't plan on buying just because it looked good and you were hungry. In one study, nearly 70 men and women were instructed to avoid eating for five hours before participating in a study in the lab. A randomly chosen half of the participants received a snack of Wheat Thins upon arrival, while the other half did not (so they remained hungry). Then they were asked to shop in a simulated online grocery store in which a higher-calorie item was displayed next to a lower-calorie item.

In a second study the researchers went to a local grocery store and tracked the purchases of over 80 people. Half of the people tracked were shopping when people are less likely to be hungry (between 1pm and 4pm) and half were shopping between 4pm and 7pm, when people are more likely to be hungry.

In the case of the online grocery store, the research team found that people bought about the same number of items whether they were hungry or not. However, those who were hungry bought more higher-calorie items - almost twice as many higher-calorie items than those who were not hungry.

In the real grocery store, those shopping in the early afternoon, when they were (presumably) not hungry, bought 4 times as many low-calorie items than high-calorie items. Shopping in the evening, however, led people to purchase more high-calorie items, bringing the ratio of low-calorie to high-calorie foods to about 2 and a half.

If you must shop when you're hungry, think ahead and make a list: then stick to it. Better yet, have a snack beforehand (a piece of fruit or some nuts). The best option, of course, is planning all your meals for the week. You can then do all your grocery shopping on one day, list in hand, and avoid the hazards of shopping while hungry completely.

1. Pre-ordering lunch at work. Results of the what to eat for lunch study. *Appetite*. 2015;84(C):88-97. doi:10.1016/j.appet.2014.10.005.
2. Byrd-Bredbenner C, Abbot JM. Differences in food supplies of U.S. households with and without overweight individuals. *Appetite*. 2009;52(2):479-484. doi:10.1016/j.appet.2008.12.011

Plan for Your Breakfast

Here are some recommendations for a good breakfast.

1. Hot Cereal with Milk (or Yogurt) and a Piece of Fruit

1/4 cup (before cooking) of oatmeal, Cream of Wheat, or grits (preferably coarse ground yellow).

2. Whole Grain Bread with Topping, a Protein, and a Piece of Fruit

Breads are best eaten with a protein. Select one from the bread choices, one topping for your bread, and one choice from the protein list.

Making muffins or quickbreads on Saturday or Sunday is a great way to have a quick, delicious breakfast on hand throughout the week. Choose higher fiber recipes. They are healthier and you'll save a lot of money over that fast food sausage biscuit.

Choose one:

1 slice of whole wheat toast

1/2 whole grain bagel (choose whole grain bagels or toast - the higher fiber, the better)

1 whole wheat English muffin

1 muffin or 1 slice quickbread from recipe

Choose one topping:

1 tsp. unsalted butter

2 tsp. preserves or jam (lower sugar versions can save you calories)

2 tsp. reduced-fat cream cheese (The "light" cream cheese is best for spreading. We use the "fat free" version mostly in baking.)

For pancakes, waffles, or French toast: 1 tsp. unsalted butter and 1 Tbsp. syrup or honey

Choose one protein:

1 large egg, cooked in as little fat as possible

2 Tbsp. peanut butter (A much better choice than other spreads.)

1 oz. low-fat cheese

1/2 cup 2% or whole milk

1 cup non-fat yogurt (Choose yogurt with no added sugar.)

3. Cold Cereal with Milk (or Yogurt) and a Piece of Fruit

Boxed cereals should have about 100 to 150 calories per serving. (All servings are one cup by volume unless noted otherwise.) Choose higher fiber and low sugar cereals.

1/2 cup of skim milk or 1% milk on your cereal is ideal. Using a half cup of non-fat yogurt is even better.

Choose one:

Cheerios (Multi-grain is best)

Kellogg's All-Bran Bran Buds (1/2 cup)

Kellogg's All-Bran Extra Fiber

Kellogg's All-Bran Original

Bite Size Shredded Wheat (not frosted)

Raisin Bran

Total Whole Grain

Total Raisin Bran

Kashi Cinnamon Harvest

Kashi GoLEAN

3. Cereal Bars

Eating a granola bar for breakfast is not a good substitute for the right breakfast. Many of them have a lot of added calories (usually as sugar) and don't include the protein that you need to help keep you satisfied through the morning.

Plan for Your Lunch

As with breakfast, a lunch "serving" should be built with a good quality carbohydrate, a protein source, and some fat. It's a good idea to pair fruit with your lunch as well. For instance, a lunch serving might be bread (mostly carbohydrates) with peanut butter (mostly protein with some fat) paired with a fruit selection.

1. Leftovers from Dinner

Dinner leftovers make the perfect lunch. It's a great idea to make extra the night before so you have something to take for lunch the next day. The rule of thumb is that a lunch serving is half of a leftover dinner serving.

For instance, if you made extra Salmon and Corn Relish today you could take the leftover dinner serving as two lunch servings.

2. Sandwiches

Whole Sandwich = 2 slices whole wheat bread with 2 ounces lean meat **or** 2 ounces reduced-fat cheese

Meat or Cheese Choices:

Leftover roasted chicken or turkey

Leftover roasted fish

2 tablespoons peanut butter

Reduced-fat Swiss cheese

Reduced-fat cheddar cheese

Reduced-fat Monterey Jack cheese

Goat cheese

Spreads:

Hellman's or Best Foods Light Mayonnaise: 1 tablespoon

Any Coarse Ground Mustard: 1 tablespoon

Dijon Style Mustard: 1 tablespoon

Your Favorite Chutney: 1 tablespoon

Roasted Garlic: 2 cloves

Toppings (as much as you want):

Sliced tomato

Lettuce

Arugula (Rocket)

Mache

Spinach

Sliced cucumber

Sliced peppers

Any kind of sprout

Cucumbers

Onions

3. Salads

Salads are a great idea! Most greens and veggies don't add up to many calories, and they are chock full of fiber, vitamins, and antioxidants. Have a salad on its own or, better yet, choose the salad and half sandwich combo.

Snack Right!

Although there's no scientific evidence that eating more frequently speeds up one's metabolism, people seem to have bought into the idea, and so snacking has become the norm. Again, there's no scientific evidence that frequent meals increase the number of calories you burn while at rest (your basal metabolism). What we do know is that often snacking simply means eating excess calories - and those excess calories can result in weight gain.

On the other hand, snacking is also sometimes compensated for by reducing the number of calories eaten at subsequent meals. Researchers in Switzerland made use of information gathered from a dietary survey of over 6,000 Swiss to look at snacking patterns as they related to weight and overall diet (1). The participants in the survey answered questions about their height and weight, whether they snacked, what they snacked on, and how often they snacked, along with questions about their diet in general. In addition they responded to demographic questions like marital status, number of children (if any), and how often they exercised.

The researchers discovered that those who snacked more frequently were no more likely to be overweight or obese than those who snacked very little. Further, those who snacked more often might have an overall healthy diet - or an unhealthy one. They did note that female respondents tended to be more health-conscious than men and tended to snack on fruit more often than men, but their overall diets tended to be healthier than men's, as well.

Snacking in and of itself is not necessarily healthy or unhealthy - it all depends on your overall diet and what you choose to snack on. If you must snack between meals, make the right choices: snacking on fruits or vegetables is a great way to get more fruits and vegetables in your diet while eating something that's low in calorie density and likely to be very satisfying because of its fiber content. Nuts are also a great snack, and we've seen studies that suggest that those added calories (in moderate amounts) won't affect your weight.

A team in Leicestershire, England noted that making those improved choices might be more satisfying for the short term, but would that higher satisfaction affect how much people ate at the next meal? (2) They recruited 12 college-age women to participate in their feeding study. All of the women had normal to slightly-above-normal Body Mass Indices, had maintained that weight for the previous six months (and were not trying to lose weight) and were screened to make sure none exhibited signs of disordered eating.

In a randomly-assigned order, each participant came to the lab on two occasions in the late afternoon and were given one of two snacks. On one occasion the snack was about 5 1/2 ounces of mixed berries (straw-berries, raspberries, blackberries, and blueberries), totaling 272 calories. On the other occasion the snack was the same number of calories but in the form of berry-flavored jelly beans. One hour after eating the snack the participants were given a standard dinner meal of pasta with tomato sauce and instructed to eat until they "were comfortably full and satisfied." If the participant consumed the entire plate of pasta, they were given another, and this was repeated until they indicated they were full. At regular intervals both before and after the snack and before and after the dinner meal the participants were asked to rate how hungry they felt along with other indications of appetite and satisfaction.

The most interesting results are that when the participants were served the berries, they ate 20% fewer calories of the later dinner meal than they did if they had the jelly beans. The researchers also note that it took the women longer to eat the berries than the candy, and after the candy snack the women ate the dinner meal more quickly. What's more, when they ate the berries as their snack, two hours after the dinner they reported feeling less hungry, more full, and having less of a desire to eat than they did when they ate the candy as a snack.

This is a very small study of all university women, so the most we can say for sure is that there is reason to perform a much larger study in a more diverse group of people. This does, however, reinforce the idea of switching to quality snacks over junk. They're definitely better for you, and they may, as this research suggests, lead you to consume fewer calories at your next meal.

The issue is, of course, that many snack foods are very calorie dense (high calories for small portions). A sweet snack like a Kit Kat bar has 220 calories and 11 grams of fat, whereas 6 Triscuits contain 120 calories and 5 grams of fat. Most such snack foods have little nutritive value.

1. Hartmann C, Siegrist M, van der Horst K. Snack frequency: associations with healthy and unhealthy food choices. *Public Health Nutr.* 2012;16(08):1487-1496. doi:10.1017/S1368980012003771.
2. James LJ, Funnell MP, Milner S. An afternoon snack of berries reduces subsequent energy intake compared to an isoenergetic confectionary snack. *Appetite.* 2015;95(C):132-137. doi:10.1016/j.appet.2015.07.005.

Hydrate Well

There is some evidence that we don't drink enough fluids throughout the day. The research is mixed, how-ever, on the optimum amount of water or other liquids that we should be consuming daily.

We know that severe dehydration can kill, with early signs of serious dehydration including confusion and delirium. Even moderate dehydration interferes with thinking processes. The studies that have investigated mild to moderate dehydration have used high temperatures as well as exercise to induce sweating enough to cause dehydration. A group at the University of Connecticut used a different approach: a combination of diuretic medications and mild exercise in 25 healthy college-age women (1).

On three separate occasions the women visited the research lab and responded to a battery of neurological tests intended to measure brain function in various areas, including memory, learning, reasoning, and mood. On one occasion the women were asked to walk on a treadmill in a moderately warm room (80F) for 40 minutes and were also given a diuretic pill to help induce dehydration. On a second occasion they performed the same exercise but were given a placebo, or sugar pill. On the third occasion they did not exercise and were also given a placebo. Before and after the tests the women's blood was tested and their urine collected to measure levels of dehydration.

The amount of exercise and the medications were designed to induce very low levels of dehydration in each participant - on the order of 1%, 2%, or 3% of total body mass - so that the researchers could assess the effects of those levels of dehydration on each participants' performance in the neurological testing.

Given that we know that serious dehydration can affect the brain, it's not surprising that the more dehydrated the women were, the poorer their scores in such areas as short-term memory, attention, and logical reasoning. What is surprising is that their moods were affected as well. The more dehydrated they were, the harder they felt a given task was to perform, the more angry or hostile they felt, and the more fatigued they felt.

This is just another reason that water should be your beverage of choice: being well hydrated can not only help keep you happier, you'll probably be more likely to feel like exercising - or continuing to exercise if you've already started. In addition to drinking water throughout the day, be sure to take a bottle of water with you when you exercise and sip on it regularly to help keep you motivated.

It appears that drinking sugar sweetened soft drinks causes weight gain and leads to an increase in the risk of diabetes. There is not a lot of research about whether drinking calorie free sodas will contribute to weight gain or not. What we do have is not encouraging for those who drink any type of soda, however.

As part of the San Antonio Heart Study, researchers in Texas looked at all soft drink consumption in a group followed for eight years (2). Of the 1,550 people who started the study, they looked at the 622 who were of clinically normal weight at the beginning of the study. The data showed that the more soft drinks of any kind that a person consumed, the more likely they were to be clinically overweight or obese. The risk is actually pretty high: for each can per day of soda (on average), the risk of developing obesity is increased by 41%. Even worse, 54% of those drinking 1 to 2 cans per day of diet drinks had become overweight during the eight years of the study.

While one should be extremely cautious in interpreting studies in animals as applying to humans, there is an interesting study where researchers at Purdue showed that rats fed artificially sweetened juices were more likely to eat more calories when presented with "regular" food (3). The researcher's interpretation was that the manipulation of sweet tastes reduced the natural ability of the rats to use sweet taste to judge the caloric content of foods they were given.

Keep in mind that humans are not rats (although we do react in similar ways to food). Whether drinking more sugar free sodas impairs the ability of humans to judge other food consumption has not been shown. There are studies, however, that show people who consume more artificial sweeteners tend to gain more weight. Keep in mind, also, that such studies as these don't prove that consuming diet drinks or artificial sweeteners **causes** weight gain - it simply shows that there is a link.

So in the end, what should you drink? Mostly water, certainly, but we know tea, green tea, and coffee are great for you. There is absolutely no evidence that coffee or tea is dangerous: neither cause high blood pressure, heart disease, or heart rhythm problems. Coffee and tea are a major source of quality antioxidants and have been shown to be beneficial in reducing the risk of diabetes.

1. Armstrong LE, Ganio MS, Casa DJ, et al. Mild Dehydration Affects Mood in Healthy Young Women. *J Nutr.* 2012;142(2):382-388. doi:10.3945/jn.111.142000
2. Scientific Sessions American Diabetic Association 2005 Abstract 1058-P
3. A Pavlovian approach to the problem of obesity, *Int J Obesity* 2004; 28: 933-935

About Coumadin®

Coumadin (warfarin) is a prescription medication used for anticoagulation. It is often referred to as "a blood thinner," but that is not really an accurate description. It works by inhibiting enzymes that lead to blood clotting. It is the only well researched, effective oral medication for this purpose. (Other brand names for warfarin are Jantoven, Marevan, and Waran.)

Its primary use is to treat or prevent blood clots. When the blood clots in a vein or artery, physicians refer to it as a thrombus. When the thrombus breaks free and travels to other parts of the body it is known as an embolus. A common problem known as deep vein thrombosis (DVT) occurs when such clots form in the large veins in the legs or arms. These will commonly form and then break free and travel to the lungs, blocking blood flow, which is known as a pulmonary embolus (PE).

Other uses include:
- ✔ Pulmonary embolism
- ✔ Artificial heart valves

- ✔ Atrial fibrillation
- ✔ Atrial flutter
- ✔ Transient ischemic attacks (TIAs)
- ✔ Stroke
- ✔ Heart attack
- ✔ Blockages of the arteries
- ✔ After some surgeries
- ✔ Those with disorders of the clotting system

How it Works

Warfarin is a synthetic version of a class of chemicals known as coumarins. These are found in many plants, including woodruff, lavender, and licorice. It was named by combining the acronym for the Wisconsin Alumni Research Foundation (WARF) and the suffix for coumarin (arin). The Foundation provided the original research grants, and it was indeed originally developed as rat poison, but is seldom used as a rat poison today because similar but much more potent forms are now available for that purpose.

Warfarin's anticoagulant effect works because the drug inhibits production of proteins known as "clotting factors." These proteins are produced in the liver and are dependent on an adequate supply of Vitamin K. The clotting factor proteins are the foundation of the "intrinsic" clotting pathway. There are many proteins that work together, and warfarin blocks four of them: Factors VII, IX, X, and II. Creation of these proteins in the liver is dependent on Vitamin K, which can come from dietary sources, but it can also be created by bacteria in the large intestine. After being absorbed, Vitamin K is stored in the liver. Consequently Vitamin K is the vital regulatory step for the production of the clotting Factors VII, IX, X, and II.

Warfarin blocks the action of Vitamin K within the liver by blocking the absorption sites in the liver needed for the uptake of Vitamin K. With the lowered ability for Vitamin K absorption, there is reduced production of the clotting factors. Consequently, dietary intake of Vitamin K affects the effectiveness of warfarin.

Prescribing Coumadin (warfarin)

Doctors prescribe Coumadin to patients who are prone to thrombosis and also to prevent thromboses in those who have already formed blood clots. There are numerous conditions that can lead to clot formation, including prosthetic heart valves, atrial fibrillation, deep venous thrombosis, and pulmonary embolism. There are also those with inherited problems with clotting factors, like antiphospholipid syndrome and factor five leiden, for whom we prescribe warfarin to prevent clotting. Sometimes the drug is used after myocardial infarction (heart attack) and stroke.

Finding the correct dose of warfarin for patients is complicated by the fact that it interacts with many other over-the-counter and prescription medications as well as supplements. This interaction can cause Coumadin to be more or less effective. The activity of the drug has to be monitored by frequent blood testing for the international normalized ratio (INR). If the INR is high, the dose of Coumadin is too high. Conversely, if the INR is too low, the medication dose needs to be increased. (Physicians used to use a test, the Prothrombin Time, sometimes called the "Pro Time" or PT, but its accuracy varied between labs. Now results are standardized through the use of the INR.)

Interactions

There are commonly used antibiotics such as erythromycin (Eryc), clarithromycin (Biaxin) and metronida-zole (Flagyl) that can markedly increase the effect of Coumadin. In some cases, using antibiotics changes the amount of the normal bacteria in the intestines and can alter the amount of Vitamin K absorbed into the body.

In addition to other medications, foods that contain higher amounts of Vitamin K also reduce the effectiveness of warfarin. To manage this, there are two basic approaches. One is to try to eat about the same amount of foods that are higher in Vitamin K each day, and the other is to completely eliminate intake of those foods that are high in Vitamin K. The latter strategy is the easier one and the one most recommended by physicians.

Genetics also play a factor in how warfarin is processed in the body. There are tests recently approved by the Food and Drug Administration that can help guide dosing of warfarin.

Adjusting the Dose

It is very important that you always know when will be your next blood test for the INR. It is equally important to know what dose you are taking. Keep a warfarin calendar to help you keep track of your dosing. Get a small calendar and carry it with you in your wallet or purse. Write your doses of warfarin in the appropriate days until the next blood test. When you take your dose, circle that day so that you know you have taken it. In the day scheduled for your blood test, write "Get INR" to remind yourself. After the test, if you have not heard from your doctor's office about your results, call them for any new instructions.

The target level of the INR will depend on why you are taking warfarin. In most cases the target range for INR is 2.0-3.0. In some cases, however, the range is higher. Your doctor will set the target based on your particular condition.

Most physicians prefer that their patients take their warfarin in the evening. This is primarily because blood tests are typically taken in the morning, and it will give your doctor time to contact you after your INR is checked. He or she can then change the dose, if needed, before you take your evening medication. There are now home testing kits available and insurance companies are paying for these more and more. Check with your doctor and your insurance company to see if you qualify.

You **must** tell **any** doctor who prescribes medicine for you that you are taking warfarin. If you have any un-usual bleeding, let your doctor know right away. Call your doctor with any questions or issues earlier rather than later. It's a good idea to have a "Medic Alert" bracelet stating that you are taking warfarin.

Common Side Effects

Rash
On rare occasions warfarin can cause a generalized rash. This has a lacy red pattern and you should call your doctor immediately to discuss this.

Bleeding
The most concerning side effect of warfarin is hemorrhage (bleeding). The risk of severe bleeding is small - on the order of 1 to 2%. In most cases where doctors prescribe warfarin, the benefit will far outweigh the risk. This is why it is so important to take care with your diet as well as being mindful of other supplements that might interact with the drug.

It may seem difficult and irritating at times for your doctor to have you get your INR level checked, but this is what allows him or her to carefully regulate the drug and reduce the risk of bleeding.

Warfarin Necrosis
A rare complication of warfarin is can be necrosis, or death of skin tissues. This happens more often in people with a deficiency of protein C.

Purple Toe Syndrome
Another rare side effect is known as purple toe syndrome. It generally occurs early after starting the medi-cation -- usually within 3 to 8 weeks. It is thought to be the result of small bits of cholesterol breaking loose from large arteries and flowing into the smaller blood vessels of the feet.

Osteoporosis
Several studies have shown a link between warfarin use and osteoporosis-related fractures.

Contraindications

Pregnant women or women who can easily become pregnant should not take warfarin. This is especially true during the first trimester, as it is known to cause deformations of the face and bones of the fetus. During the third trimester there is a high risk of bleeding. There are alternatives such as heparin, however.

Other Interactions

Taking other medications can also increase the risk of bleeding. The most common are antiplatelet drugs such as aspirin, clopidogrel or nonsteroidal anti-inflammatory drugs like ibuprofen (Advil) or naproxyn (Aleve, Naprosyn).

There are many other drug-to-drug interactions, and because of genetic factors the body's processing of the drug can vary widely between patients.

Excessive alcohol use can also affect how warfarin is processed in the liver and elevate the INR. Most physicians will caution patients about the use of alcohol while taking warfarin. Commonly doctors will allow a few drinks after INR is stable.

Foods that are high in Vitamin K have also been reported to interact with warfarin. See the list at the end of this book for a list of commonly-consumed foods.

Supplements

Warfarin also interacts with many herbs, including (but not limited to):
- ✔ Ginkgo Biloba
- ✔ St. John's Wort
- ✔ American Ginseng
- ✔ Garlic as a supplement (not fresh garlic)

Vitamin K Dosage

I get the question all the time about how much Vitamin K is right for folks taking Coumadin (warfarin). Unfortunately, there's no perfect study to guide just how much Vitamin K is too much for those taking Coumadin. Most physicians recommend limiting foods that contain very high or even moderate amounts of Vitamin K. At the same time, there's never been a recommendation to severely limit Vitamin K intake.

The Recommended Daily Allowance (RDA) for Vitamin K is about 80 micrograms (mcg) for males and 70 mcg for females. The majority of ingredients contain small amounts - in the under 15 mcg range - so keeping an eye on foods that contain more than 20 - 25 mcg per serving is a good rule of thumb.

Avoiding **all** Vitamin K might be just as much of a problem as getting too much, however. Studies have clearly shown that eating foods that are higher in Vitamin K will have an effect on the effectiveness of Coumadin and the INR. Most people who either take warfarin themselves or those who help patients manage their anti-coagulation know this, but there is some research now that shows eating **too little** Vitamin K can have the same effect.

So what to do? How much is too much? How little is too little? It appears, from what research we have, that in those folks who were taking Coumadin, 29 mcg was too little and 76 mcg just right to keep their INR stable.

While it's not a perfect way to look at the issue of how much is too much Vitamin K in the diet for warfarin users, another study showed an effect on the INR in those taking 150 - 200 mcg per day in Vitamin K supplements. These are the levels found in Vitamin K rich foods such as spinach, collard greens and broccoli.

For the number of folks who use this medication and the fact that there's no great replacement on the horizon, it is a shame that a large study has not been done to help answer this question more clearly. For the time being, we have to be content with the small studies that point toward an optimum near the RDA guidelines for Vitamin K.

Frequently Asked Questions About Warfarin

Q: Does salt increase INR levels?

My girlfriend (age 46) just had a heart valve replacement and was placed on Coumadin. She was told to avoid food with a high sodium content. We have some questions about this and what actually affect her INR levels.

Does salt actually increase the INR level? They also told her she could use "sea salt" in moderation, but from what I have read it's still salt, is this true? Is sea salt really better for you?

What about the lack of iodine in sea salt, I have not found any iodized sea salt yet. Does she need to worry about iodine supplements if using non-iodized sea salt or salt substitutes?

A: The sodium content of table salt (sodium chloride) should not have an effect on your girlfriend's INR or her Coumadin® (warfarin). It may be that her doctor wanted to make sure that there are no problems with salt worsening her high blood pressure or issues of fluid overload in the body that could lead to Congestive Heart Failure (CHF).

Sea salt is salt. A teaspoon might have a little less sodium in it because of the fact that sea salt crystals are larger and therefore don't stack together in a spoon like Morton's salt. That said, salt is salt. There are impurities in sea salt that can contribute to flavors in the salt, but otherwise the sodium and chloride are the same. Sea salt is salt and all salt in excess is something that pretty much everyone should avoid. I don't see that sea salt is worth the extra money.

Most folks get enough iodine in a healthy diet. Using a mixture of salt and sea salt should be fine, but check with her doctor about the amount of sodium he wants her to have each day. She really shouldn't need to worry about iodine supplements this way.

Q: Can I cook with parsley while on Coumadin?

I am trying to work out my new diet. The list says 1 cup of raw parsley is very high. Can I use a small amount to cook with?

A: There's a good chance that parsley accounts for most of the variation that physicians and patients find with INR levels in those taking Coumadin (warfarin).

This is because parsley contains a lot of Vitamin K. The USDA Ingredient Database reports that just a tablespoon has 62 micrograms (mcg). This can add up quite fast in a meal that has a couple of tablespoons of parsley as a garnish or in a dressing. It would be best to be very cautious unless you know exactly how much Vitamin K is in a particular dish (including the parsley).

Q: Should I avoid lettuce while on Coumadin?

I was told that if you are on Coumadin you should not eat lettuce. Is this true?

A: Because Vitamin K can have an effect on how Coumadin® (warfarin) is processed in your body it is important to have about the same amounts of Vitamin K each day.

Lettuces are members of the cabbage family. As a rule cabbages contain higher amounts of Vitamin K. Part of eating healthy is to eat a lot of green leafy vegetables, but this can be a problem for those people who use Coumadin as a result. If you are going to begin eating lettuce and other members of the cabbage family, it is important to be **consistent.** By that I mean you should eat about the same amount of such green leafy vegetables each day so that your INR doesn't fluctuate.

Take a look at the Vitamin K Levels in Foods list later in this book. Take this to your doctor and discuss eating a consistent daily serving of such foods. That way the two of you can more closely monitor your INR while you are adapting your diet.

Q: Can you wean down your dose of Coumadin?

Is it possible to increase certain things like Vitamin E, A, and C so that you can lower the dose of Coumadin needed? Of course you would have to be monitored by your doctor, but is it possible to use garlic or some natural ways to thin your blood so you would not have to take so much Coumadin?

I'm a registered nurse and my cousin has to take 30 pills every day, including 10mg of Coumadin. She is asking me if there is any way she could be weaned off of some of the medicine. Besides lowering her intake of Vitamin K what else can she do to thin her blood?

A: We don't know of any research that supports using vitamins or other supplements to reduce the dose of Coumadin® (warfarin). Often a visit with the patient's doctor to discuss reducing and consolidating medications can be helpful.

There are **no clinically proven methods** to help "thin" her blood other than the medications recommended by her physician.

Q: Does Coumadin cause fatigue?

My mother is on Coumadin. She is also on Vicodin for pain. She is chronically tired all the time! Is Coumadin a contributing factor for this tiredness? I know that the Vicodin is. Can you help me know what foods she could eat to boost her energy?

A: Your question is a common one. Certainly the Vicodin can be a major contributing factor to your mother's fatigue, and using narcotics in the elderly for pain control can be a challenge.

Fatigue is not, however, a common complaint of those using Coumadin® (warfarin), but we know that patients will react to medications in different ways - so it is possible that your mother's tiredness is related. There may be other medications that could be causing issues. For example, there are common medications that some take while taking Coumadin that might be involved. These include beta blockers (atenolol, metoprolol, propranolol, etc.), calcium channel blockers (amlodipine, diltiazem) as well as many antidepressants.

Often depression can be the culprit and depression should always be considered when treating fatigue in the elderly. Part of the work up for fatigue and depression includes evaluating thyroid function and Vitamin

B12 levels, and hemoglobin is key in the work up for fatigue as well. Chat with your mother about going with her to the next doctor's appointment. Many times our elderly patients will tell their physicians "everything's just fine" when it isn't. Many doctors have heard their patients say, "I just didn't want to bother you with my problems -- you need to take your time with someone who is really sick." (Except, of course, it's your mother who we want to take care of.)

There is a great deal of controversy about whether foods can boost energy or not. Certainly there are thousands of websites claiming that particular foods and diets can provide everything from energy to longevity to boosting the immune system. While much of the research that has been done is encouraging regarding the effect of diet on long term health, most are smaller studies and require more research. Likewise, few have shown specific short term benefits for malaise and fatigue.

That said, diet is often a concern. A major issue in the elderly can be that they will often not cook fresh foods for themselves and sometimes eat less healthy. Skipping meals can be a major problem, as well as relying on more processed foods and not getting fresh, whole foods. The consequence can be fewer calories than they actually need and the quality of those calories can be lacking.

One strategy is to ask her if you can take a look in her cabinets and fridge. Sometimes the food is there but she might not be eating it. Having your mom keep a food diary can be one path to seeing what she is eating and how often.

Lastly, there are many local and community services that will help provide her with ready made meals. Resources include acl.gov/ltc as well as www.nia.nih.gov/health/aging-place-growing-older-home

Q: Does Coumadin® (warfarin) cause weight gain?

My wife has been taking warfarin for over two months. When she started exercising for three days a week, in a month's time she has gained 12 pounds, and her diet did not change. Before she started exercising she was losing some amount of weight. She will be using warfarin for the next four months. Do you think warfarin has affected her metabolism? If yes how could she lose weight then?

A: This is a very interesting question. There is no evidence that Coumadin (warfarin) leads to weight gain. As a physician my first question would be whether there is a medical issue that is leading to your wife's weight gain. It is important that she discuss this with her doctor. Perhaps there is another medication that she is taking that could lead to weight gain. Some people who take Coumadin for certain heart problems are more susceptible to congestive heart failure and that is the sort of issue her physician would want to know about.

Weight loss is accomplished by eating fewer calories and exercising more. Often people will use supplements like sports drinks and the like while exercising that they feel are healthy but are actually just added calories. Keeping a food diary is a good first step for your wife. This can help her to get an idea of what she is eating. Many times asking one's doctor for a referral to the dietician can help and having the food diary can be an aid to helping create a diet that works for your wife.

Q: Should you avoid cranberry juice on Coumadin® (warfarin)?

My husband may have a kidney infection and I wanted to give him cranberry juice, but he is on Coumadin. Would this affect his medicine?

A: Up until recently I would have said that it would be wise to avoid it. A report in the *British Medical Journal* in 2003 was concerning. The patient in question was drinking a great deal of cranberry juice and on an essentially liquid diet. There were other case reports, but no well-designed study that investigated the issue until more recently. The good news is that we now have pretty good evidence that it's OK to drink cranberry juice.

The feeling had been that somehow cranberry juice interacted with the cytochrome P450 system of enzymes, which are critical to helping the body clear itself of chemicals such as medications we take.

A group of researchers in Boston looked at whether cranberry juice, brewed tea, grape juice or placebo would have an effect on the specific P450 enzyme responsible for clearing warfarin from the body. They used another drug, fluconazole, as a control medication. (*Clin Pharmacol Ther* 2006;79:125-33.) No effect was seen on the clearance of medications in the body by any of the test substances.

In another study, a group had ten healthy volunteers drink cranberry juice or water each day for ten days. They tested three different drugs, including warfarin, to see if there was any difference in the drug concentrations or the INR. Again, no difference. (*Clin Pharmacol Ther* 2007;81:833-39.) We were right to be cautious because of the case reports, but now we have evidence that it's OK for you to drink cranberry juice while taking Coumadin (warfarin).

Q: Does alcohol interact with Coumadin?

My mother is taking Coumadin. For years when my brother comes over for Monday night dinner my mom and brother have one shot of Crown Royal. Could my mom have a tiny bite of alcohol? If she does, what will happen? She is 91 years old.

A: Most physicians deal with alcohol use in their patients on a case by case basis.

The amount of Crown Royal is small enough that it would likely not be a problem for your mom's warfarin use. However, patients who take Coumadin are often on a number of other medications that alcohol can interact with.

Check with her doctor to make sure that he or she feels a drink with your Monday night dinners is OK.

Q: Should I avoid caffeinated coffee on Coumadin® (warfarin)?

I am on Coumadin, do I have to drink Decaf coffee only. If I drink regular coffee, would it give me a headache?

A: Many physicians wish for their patients to not consume caffeine. There is scant evidence to support this posture, but many people do feel better drinking coffee or tea with no caffeine. You would need to ask your doctor how he or she feels about this for your case.

Many people who drink a lot of beverages that contain caffeine develop a dependency. When they stop consuming caffeine abruptly they can often have symptoms of fatigue and headache. If you are used to drinking a lot of regular coffee, it might be a good idea for you to taper off slowly, drinking a little less each day for about a week.

One way to do this is to mix regular coffee with decaf before you brew the coffee. Each day use less regular and more decaf in brewing. After a week or so you will be using only decaffeinated.

Q: How much Vitamin K is in Fresca®, Sprite®, or other sodas?

Hello-my father is on Coumadin (almost died of a AAA). We were discussing that his levels fluctuate because of Fresca soda or maybe some Sprite/7Up he drinks. Would this have a major factor on his med. Also when you discuss Cola-does root beer fall in this category.

A: The USDA reports that Sprite® contains no Vitamin K at all. Their database doesn't contain information on Fresca® but there is information on many other types of soda. Cola, with or without caffeine as well as with or without sugar, does not have any Vitamin K.

The same is true for cream soda, club soda, ginger ale, grape soda, Dr. Pepper®, orange soda, root beer and tonic water.

It appears that users of Coumadin® (warfarin) would be safe drinking soda. That said, soda is not a good choice for a healthy diet. Drinking a cola or root beer occasionally is fine and one should choose sugar free products. There is plenty of research now that shows how much better other beverages can be for your health. Choose water, juice, tea, coffee, or green tea instead.

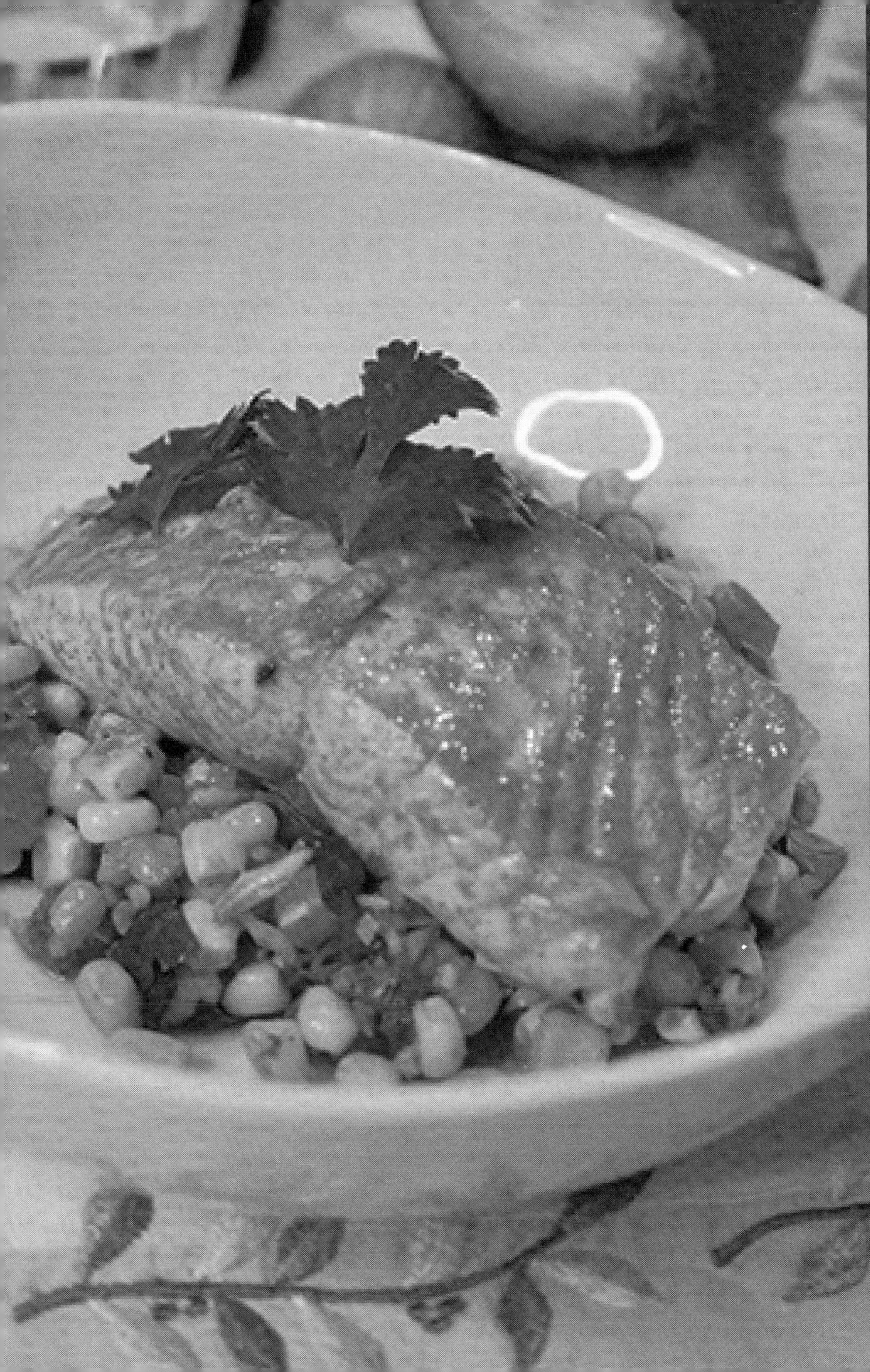

Apple Pancake

Servings: 4 | Serving size: 1/4 pancake

Cooking time: 30 minutes

To multiply this recipe it's best to make two separate batches in two skillets. Leftovers are actually pretty good. Wrap tightly after cooled and refrigerate.

2 lbs. (4 medium)	granny smith apples
2 tsp.	unsalted butter
1/2 cup	Splenda or stevia
1/4 cup	water
3	large egg whites
1	large egg yolk
3/4 cup	non-fat buttermilk
3/4 cup	all purpose flour
1/4 tsp.	salt
2 Tbsp.	Splenda or stevia
2 tsp.	unsalted butter

Peel and core apples. Discard the peel. Slice very thin (about 1/8 inch thick).

Preheat oven to 425°F.

In a 12 inch iron skillet (or non-stick skillet) heat the butter, Splenda and water until boiling. Add apples and cook about 15 minutes. Stir the apples gently about every 3 minutes. As the apples cook the liquid will reduce and the mixture will turn a light golden brown caramel color. The bottom of the apples should be a caramel brown.

While the apples are cooking place the egg whites, egg yolk, buttermilk, flour, salt and the 2 tablespoons Splenda in a blender. Blend until smooth.

When the apples are caramelized pour the flour/buttermilk mixture over the apples so that the liquid covers them completely.

Transfer the pan to the oven and bake for about 15 - 18 minutes. The pancake is done when it is brown on top. It will puff slightly as it cooks.
Remove from the oven and place the 2 tsp. butter on top of the pancake to melt.

The refrigerator light goes on...
A dish like this one is perfect for a special occasion brunch. The best part is that if there are leftovers, they make good desserts a day or two later.

Nutrition Facts	
Serving size	1/4 pie
Servings	`4
Calories 205	Calories from Fat 50
	% Daily Value
Total Fat 6 g	9 %
Saturated Fat 3 g	16 %
Trans Fat 0 g	
Monounsaturated Fat 2 g	
Cholesterol 64 mg	21 %
Sodium 237 mg	10 %
Total Carbohydrates 31 g	10 %
Dietary Fiber 2 g	10 %
Sugars 11 g	
Protein 8 g	
Vitamin A 4 %	Vitamin C 6 %
Calcium 7 %	Iron 7 %
Vitamin K 1 mcg	
Potassium 218 mg	
Magnesium 17 mg	

Blueberry Muffins

Servings: 6 | Serving size: 1 muffin

Cooking time: 30 minutes

This recipe can be multiplied by 2. Muffins will keep for 24 - 36 hours in a plastic bag. These freeze fairly well if sealed tightly in a plastic bag.

2 tsp	canola oil
1/2 cup	Splenda or stevia
1 large	egg
2 Tbsp	non-fat yogurt
1/2 tsp	pure vanilla extract
1 cup	all purpose white flour
1/2 cup	whole wheat flour
2 Tbsp	wheat germ
1/4 tsp	salt
1 tsp	baking powder
1/4 tsp	baking soda
1/2 cup	low-fat buttermilk
1/2 cup	blueberries

Preheat oven to 375°F.

Separate the egg into an egg white and egg yolk. Set the egg yolk aside and whisk the egg white until frothy.

Cream together the canola oil and egg yolk until smooth. Add the Z-Sweet or Splenda®, yogurt and vanilla extract.

Whisk until smooth.

Place the all-purpose flour, whole wheat flour, wheat germ, salt, baking powder and baking soda in a sifter and sift into the mixing bowl.

Gently fold the creamed mixture together with the flour mixture. As this is blended slowly add the buttermilk folding until smooth. As soon as the mixture is well blended, stop.

Fold the frothed egg white into the batter. Gently fold the blueberries into the batter. Do not over mix.

Line a muffin tin with muffin papers and fill each muffin paper with an equal amount of batter. Bake for 12 - 15 minutes.

The refrigerator light goes on...
This is a great muffin that's so much better for you than a regular muffin. When I started with Dr. Gourmet I wanted to make food that people found familiar but healthier. This takes that a step further than the previous Blueberry Muffins posted on the web site because of the higher fiber content. One taster said that these "are so much better tasting than the original." That's what great food is -- good food that just happens to be better for you.

Nutrition Facts	
Serving size	1 muffin
Servings	6
Calories 163	Calories from Fat 27
	% Daily Value
Total Fat 3 g	5 %
Saturated Fat 1 g	3 %
Trans Fat 0 g	
Monounsaturated Fat 2 g	
Cholesterol 36 mg	12 %
Sodium 265 mg	11 %
Total Carbohydrates 28 g	9 %
Dietary Fiber 2 g	10 %
Sugars 3 g	
Protein 6 g	
Vitamin A 1 %	Vitamin C 2 %
Calcium 9 %	Iron 10 %
Vitamin K 4 mcg	
Potassium 134 mg	
Magnesium 29 mg	

Scrambled Eggs

Servings: 2 | Serving size: 2 eggs

Cooking time: 30 minutes

This recipe can easily be multiplied by 2. Scrambled Eggs keep O.K. for about 24 hours and make great sandwiches with a bit of mayo, lettuce and tomato.

3	large egg whites
1	large egg yolk
2 Tbsp.	water
1/8 tsp.	salt
1 tsp.	unsalted butter
8 ounces	fresh crimini mushrooms (sliced)
to taste	fresh ground black pepper

Place the egg whites, egg yolk, water and salt in a small mixing bowl and whisk until frothy.

Melt the butter in a small non-stick skillet pan over medium-high heat. Gently sauté the mushrooms until browned. Toss frequently. Cook the mushrooms until they are a dark caramel brown.

Add egg mixture and stir the eggs cooking until firm.

Add fresh ground black pepper to taste and serve.

The refrigerator light goes on...
Eggs are good for you. Period. Quit worrying and enjoy them. You can substitute almost any veggie for the mushrooms. Scrambled eggs are especially good with red or green bell peppers.

Nutrition Facts	
Serving size	2 eggs
Servings	2
Calories 96	Calories from Fat 45
	% Daily Value
Total Fat 5 g	7 %
Saturated Fat 2 g	11 %
Trans Fat 0 g	
Monounsaturated Fat 2 g	
Cholesterol 110 mg	37 %
Sodium 383 mg	16 %
Total Carbohydrates 4 g	1 %
Dietary Fiber 1 g	4 %
Sugars 2 g	
Protein 10 g	
Vitamin A 4 %	Vitamin C 4 %
Calcium 2 %	Iron 5 %
Vitamin K 0 mcg	
Potassium 447 mg	
Magnesium 16 mg	

Blueberry Pancakes

Servings: 2 | Serving size: 2 pancakes

Cooking time: 30 minutes

This recipe can be halved or multiplied by 2 or 3. Leftover pancakes aren't very good. The batter will keep overnight but the pancakes will not be as good.

6 Tbsp.	whole wheat flour
6 Tbsp.	all purpose flour
3 Tbsp.	medium grind yellow corn meal
1/8 tsp.	salt
1 tsp.	baking powder
1 tsp.	sugar
6 Tbsp.	old fashioned oatmeal
1 cup	non-fat buttermilk
1	large egg
2	large egg whites
1/2 cup	blueberries
2 tsp./serving	unsalted butter
1 Tbsp./serving	pure maple syrup

Sift the whole wheat flour, all purpose whole wheat flour, all purpose flour, corn meal, salt, baking powder and sugar into a large mixing bowl.

Fold in the oatmeal.

Add the buttermilk and eggs and blend well until mixture is smooth.

Heat a non-stick griddle over medium-high heat.

Let the batter stand for at least 2 minutes while the griddle is heating.

Stir once and wait another minute before placing batter on the griddle.

When the griddle is hot enough that a few drops of water will dance on the surface, reduce the heat to medium and place about 1/4 cup of batter for each pancake on the griddle.

Top with the blueberries.

Cook until small bubbles on the surface of the pan-cake form and then burst.

Turn and cook for about 1/2 the time that the pancakes cooked on the first side.

Remove and top with butter and maple syrup.

The refrigerator light goes on...
I love adding fruit to my pancakes. Any berry will do -- blueberries, strawberries, blackberries -- whatever is in the market. I have not had much success using frozen berries in my pancakes, however.

Nutrition Facts	
Serving size	2 pancakes with butter and maple syrup
Servings	2
Calories 460	Calories from Fat 108
	% Daily Value
Total Fat 12 g	16 %
Saturated Fat 6 g	30 %
Trans Fat 0 g	
Monounsaturated Fat 3.5 g	
Cholesterol 115 mg	38 %
Sodium 490 mg	21 %
Total Carbohydrates 75 g	27 %
Dietary Fiber 6 g	23 %
Sugars 18 g	
Protein 15 g	
Vitamin A 12 %	Vitamin C 4 %
Calcium 15 %	Iron 21 %
Vitamin K 9 mcg	
Potassium 400 mg	
Magnesium 75 mg	

Jean's French Toast

Servings: 2 | Serving size: 2 slices bread

Cooking time: 30 minutes

This recipe can easily be halved or doubled. Left-over French Toast is not very good. This batter doesn't keep well.

2 large	eggs
1 tsp.	sugar
6 Tbsp.	2% milk
1/4 tsp.	ground nutmeg
1/2 tsp.	pure vanilla extract
3 tsp.	unsalted butter
4 - 1 ounce slices	sourdough bread
2 Tbsp.	pure maple syrup

Place the egg, sugar, milk, ground nutmeg and vanilla in a large mixing bowl.

Whisk until well blended.

Heat a non-stick griddle over medium-high heat.

When the griddle is hot enough that a few drops of water will dance on the surface, reduce the heat to medium and place 4 slices of bread into the batter.

Gently dunk and turn the bread until it is well coated and slightly soaked.

Place the 4 slices of soaked bread on the griddle and cook for about 3 – 4 minutes.

Turn and cook on the other side.

Cook, turning occasionally, until both sides are golden brown.

Depending on your stove or griddle you may need to reduce the heat slightly.

Remove and top with one teaspoon of butter on each piece of toast and serve with pure maple syrup.

The refrigerator light goes on...
This French Toast is based on an old family recipe. The amazing thing about this recipe is the nutmeg. Most French Toast recipes use cinnamon, but the ground nutmeg creates a much more elegant flavor.

Nutrition Facts	
Serving size	2 slices French Toast w/1 tsp. unsalted butter and 1 Tbsp. pure maple syrup
Servings	2
Calories 290	Calories from Fat 56
	% Daily Value
Total Fat 8 g	10 %
Saturated Fat 2.5 g	13 %
Trans Fat 0 g	
Monounsaturated Fat 2.5 g	
Cholesterol 185 mg	62 %
Sodium 370 mg	16 %
Total Carbohydrates 42 g	15 %
Dietary Fiber <1 g	3 %
Sugars 15 g	
Protein 8 g	
Vitamin A 9 %	Vitamin C 0 %
Calcium 5 %	Iron 15 %
Vitamin K 0 mcg	
Potassium 200 mg	

Zucchini and Chévre Frittata

Servings: 2 | Serving size: 1/2 pie

Cooking time: 30 minutes

This recipe can be multiplied by 2 but requires a larger skillet. Leftovers are good. Wrap tightly after cooled and refrigerate. I like to make sandwiches from left over frittata.

1 medium	zucchini (sliced thin length-wise)
	olive oil spray
1 tsp.	unsalted butter
1 clove	garlic (minced)
1/2	red onion (sliced)
2	large eggs
2	large egg whites
2 Tbsp.	water
1/8 tsp.	salt
2 Tbsp.	Parmigiano-Reggiano (grated)
1 ounce	semi soft goat cheese
to taste	fresh ground black pepper

Preheat the oven to 425°F.

Place the zucchini on a non-stick cookie sheet and lightly spray with olive oil. Place the cookie sheet in the oven and roast the zucchini for about 7 – 10 minutes turning once. Remove and cool.

Heat 1/2 teaspoon butter in a small non-stick skillet over low-medium heat and add the garlic. Increase the heat and cook slowly over medium heat stirring frequently. Do not allow the garlic to brown. Add the sliced red onion and continue to cook until translucent. Set aside.

Whisk the eggs, egg whites, water and salt in a bowl until frothy. Fold in the Parmigiano-Reggiano.

Heat the remaining butter in a small non-stick skillet over high heat and when bubbling add the egg mixture. Reduce the heat to medium and simmer for about 2 minutes. Add the onion/garlic mixture distributing it across the top of the eggs.

Layer the zucchini slices on top in a crisscross pattern and then crumble the goat cheese over the top of the zucchini. Grind fresh pepper on top to taste.

Place in oven and cook for about 15 minutes until it puffs and is firm to the touch.

The refrigerator light goes on...
Just a little bit of rich cheese makes for a wonderfully rich recipe but doesn't add many calories.

Nutrition Facts		
Serving size		1/2 pie
Servings		2
Calories 211	Calories from Fat 113	
		% Daily Value
Total Fat 13 g		20 %
Saturated Fat 7 g		33 %
Trans Fat 0 g		
Monounsaturated Fat 4 g		
Cholesterol 237 mg		79 %
Sodium 425 mg		18 %
Total Carbohydrates 9 g		3 %
Dietary Fiber 2 g		7 %
Sugars 4 g		
Protein 17 g		18 %
Vitamin A 15 %	Vitamin C 33 %	
Calcium 15 %	Iron 9 %	
Vitamin K 5 mcg		
Potassium 467 mg		
Magnesium 36 mg		

Polenta and Eggs

Servings: 1 | Serving Size: 1 cup polenta and one egg

Cooking time: 30 minutes

This recipe can easily be multiplied but does not make very good leftovers.

1 cup	water
1/4 cup	coarse ground cornmeal (aka polenta or grits)
1/8 tsp	salt
to taste	fresh ground black pepper
1 large	egg
1 Tbsp	Parmigiano-Reggiano (grated)

Preheat the oven to 375°F.

Place the water in a small sauce pan over high heat.

When the water is boiling, whisk in the polenta. Add it gradually while whisking so that it doesn't clump.

Add the salt and pepper to the pan.

Reduce the heat to medium so that the polenta is simmering. Whisk almost continuously. After about 5 minutes, the polenta should be about the thickness of house paint.

Pour the polenta into a shallow dish, like an au gratin dish or even a small soufflé dish.

Crack the egg and pour it in the middle of the polenta. Place the dish in the oven and bake for 5 minutes. Sprinkle the parmesan over the top and cook for another 3 to 5 minutes.

Serve.

The refrigerator light goes on...
Eggs are great for you and this is a great way to have them. It's sort of like toad in the hole with great flavorful carbs and rich yummy eggs.

Nutrition Facts	
Serving size	1 cup polenta and 1 egg
Servings	1
Calories 189	Calories from Fat 58
	% Daily Value
Total Fat 7 g	10 %
Saturated Fat 2 g	10 %
Trans Fat 0 g	
Monounsaturated Fat 2 g	
Cholesterol 41 mg	14 %
Sodium 400 mg	17 %
Total Carbohydrates 24 g	8 %
Dietary Fiber 2 g	9 %
Sugars 1 g	
Protein 9 g	
Vitamin A 6 %	Vitamin C 0 %
Calcium 5 %	Iron 11 %
Vitamin K 1 mcg	
Potassium 156 mg	

Four Grain Pancakes

Servings: 2 | Serving size: 2 pancakes

Cooking time: 30 minutes

This recipe can be halved or multiplied by 2 or 3. Leftover pancakes aren't very good. The batter will keep overnight but the pancakes will not be as good.

6 Tbsp.	whole wheat flour
6 Tbsp.	all purpose flour
3 Tbsp.	medium grind yellow corn meal
1/8 tsp.	salt
1 tsp.	baking powder
1 Tbsp.	Z-sweet stevia or Splenda
6 Tbsp.	old fashioned oatmeal
1 cup	non-fat buttermilk
1	large egg
2	large egg whites
2 tsp. (per serving)	unsalted butter
1 Tbsp. (per serving)	pure maple syrup

Sift the whole wheat flour, all purpose flour, corn meal, salt, baking powder, and sweetener into a large mixing bowl.

Fold in the oatmeal.

Add the buttermilk, egg, and egg whites, and blend well until mixture is smooth.

Heat a non-stick griddle over medium-high heat. Let the batter stand for at least 2 minutes while the griddle is heating. Stir once and wait another minute before placing batter on the griddle.

When the griddle is hot enough that a few drops of water will dance on the surface, reduce the heat to medium and place about 1/4 cup of batter for each pancake on the griddle.

Cook until small bubbles on the surface of the pancake form and then burst. Turn and cook for about 1/2 the time that the pancakes cooked on the first side.

Remove and top with one teaspoon of unsalted butter on each pancake and serve one tablespoon of pure maple syrup for every two pancakes.

The refrigerator light goes on...
These are really good for you with tons of fiber, but because of the calories, best saved for a late Sunday brunch. You can also use flavored syrup.

Nutrition Facts	
Serving size	2 pancakes, w/2 tsp. unsalted butter and 1 Tbsp. pure maple syrup
Servings	2
Calories 437	Calories from Fat 70
	% Daily Value
Total Fat 8 g	2 %
Saturated Fat 2 g	12 %
Trans Fat 0 g	
Monounsaturated Fat 3 g	
Cholesterol 107 mg	36 %
Sodium 469 mg	20 %
Total Carbohydrates 76 g	25 %
Dietary Fiber 6 g	24 %
Sugars 19 g	
Protein 17 g	
Vitamin A 18 %	Vitamin C 2 %
Calcium 34 %	Iron 20 %
Vitamin K 4 mcg	
Potassium 482 mg	
Magnesium 89 mg	

Tortilla

Servings: 4 | Serving size: 1/4 pie

Cooking time: 60 minutes

This recipe can be multiplied by 2 but requires a larger skillet. This recipe keeps well for about 24 – 48 hours and is good both cold and hot.

3 quarts	water
3/4 lb.	red potatoes
8	large egg whites
2	large egg yolks
1 Tbsp.	fresh curly or flat leaf parsley (minced)
1/4 tsp.	salt
2 tsp.	fresh oregano (chopped)
1/8 tsp.	red pepper flakes
1/2 tsp.	jalapeño (seeded and minced)
to taste	fresh ground black pepper
2 tsp.	extra virgin olive oil
1	medium white onion (diced)

Place the water in medium stock pot over high heat and bring to a boil. Reduce the heat to medium-high and cook the potatoes until slightly tender (about 20 minutes). Drain and let the potatoes cool slightly. Cut into 1/2 inch cubes.

Preheat the oven to 350°F.

Whisk together the egg whites, egg yolks, parsley, salt, oregano, red pepper flakes and minced jalapeño. Add fresh ground pepper to taste and then add the potatoes. Fold together gently until well blended.

Heat the olive oil in a 10 inch non-stick skillet over high heat and add the onions. Cook, stirring continuously, until soft and golden brown. Reduce the heat to medium and add the eggs/potato mixture.

Cook two minutes on the stove and then transfer to the oven and cook for about twenty minutes (until the center is set).

The refrigerator light goes on...

This dish is great right out of the oven but is even better the next day after it has chilled. This is the most common way that it is served in Spain and can be found all over the country in Tapas bars. Because the tortilla is made with eggs, be careful to keep it well chilled before serving.

The word tortilla comes from the latin root word torte which means cake. The flat unleavened bread (cake) that we know as a tortilla is the accompaniment for (or major ingredient of) many Mexican recipes.

The tortilla that is served in Spain is a baked omelet (cake="torta") usually made with potatoes. It is mildly spiced and often served at room temperature. The tortilla is similar to the Italian frittata (which usually doesn't use potatoes in the recipe).

Nutrition Facts	
Serving size	1/4 pie
Servings	4
Calories 153	Calories from Fat 43
	% Daily Value
Total Fat 5 g	7 %
Saturated Fat 1 g	6 %
Trans Fat 0 g	
Monounsaturated Fat 3 g	
Cholesterol 105 mg	35 %
Sodium 266 mg	11 %
Total Carbohydrates 17 g	6 %
Dietary Fiber 2 g	8 %
Sugars 3 g	
Protein 11 g	
Vitamin A 5 %	Vitamin C 18 %
Calcium 4 %	Iron 6 %
Vitamin K 21 mcg	
Potassium 551 mg	
Magnesium 30 mg	

Orange French Toast

Servings: 2 | Serving size: 2 slices toast

Cooking time: 30 minutes

This recipe can easily be doubled. Leftover French Toast is not very good. This batter doesn't keep well.

French Toast

1 large	egg
2 tsp.	Grand Marnier orange liqueur
1/2 tsp.	sugar
1 Tbsp.	2% milk
1/4 tsp.	pure vanilla extract
1/4 cup	orange juice
1/4 tsp.	orange zest
4 slices	sourdough bread
2 tsp. (per serving)	unsalted butter

Orange Honey

2 Tbsp.	honey
1/2 tsp.	Grand Marnier orange liqueur

Place the egg, Grand Marnier, sugar, milk, vanilla extract, orange juice, and orange zest in a medium-mixing bowl. Whisk until well blended.

Heat a non-stick griddle over medium-high heat.

When the griddle is hot enough that a few drops of water will dance on the surface, reduce the heat to medium and place 4 slices of bread into the batter. Gently dunk and turn the bread until it is well coated and slightly soaked.

Place the 4 slices of soaked bread on the griddle and cook for about 3 - 4 minutes. Turn and cook on the other side.

Cook, turning occasionally, until both sides are golden brown. Depending on your stove or griddle, you may need to reduce the heat slightly.

Remove and top with one teaspoon of unsalted butter on each piece of toast and serve one tablespoon of orange honey for every two slices of French toast.

The refrigerator light goes on...
French Toast itself isn't all that bad for you and a great treat for Sunday morning brunch. Enriched sauces, such as Orange Honey, can add different flavors to your pancakes or French toast.

Nutrition Facts	
Serving size	2 slices French Toast
	w/2 tsp. unsalted butter
	and 1 Tbsp. orange honey
Servings	2
Calories 350	Calories from Fat 81
	% Daily Value
Total Fat 9 g	12 %
Saturated Fat 5 g	26 %
Trans Fat 0 g	
Monounsaturated Fat 2.5 g	
Cholesterol 20 mg	7 %
Sodium 410 mg	18 %
Total Carbohydrates 57 g	21 %
Dietary Fiber 2 g	6 %
Sugars 26 g	
Protein 9 g	
Vitamin A 8 %	Vitamin C 18 %
Calcium 3 %	Iron 15 %
Vitamin K 1 mcg	
Potassium 200 mg	

Orange Blueberry Scones

Servings: 8 | Serving size: 1 scone

Cooking time: 30 minutes

This recipe doesn't multiply well. The scones will keep sealed in plastic for about 36 hours. If refrigerated, they should also be sealed in plastic, and will keep for 96 hours.

2 cups	all purpose flour
1/4 cup	light brown sugar
2 tsp.	baking powder
1/2 tsp.	salt
2 Tbsp.	unsalted butter (softened)
1 tsp.	fresh grated orange peel
1/4 cup	orange juice
3/4 cup	non-fat buttermilk
1/4 cup	blueberries
2 Tbsp.	non-fat buttermilk
1 Tbsp.	light brown sugar

Preheat oven to 425°F.

Sift the flour, brown sugar, baking powder and salt into a large mixing bowl.

Cut in the softened butter with the tines of a fork or a pastry knife. It is well blended when the mixture is the consistency of coarse corn meal.

Add the orange juice and orange peel slowly while kneading the batter (I use a rubber spatula). Continue kneading while adding the buttermilk. The mixture will become a sticky dough.

Gently fold in the blueberries taking care not to let any burst.

Divide the dough into eight small triangles onto a non-stick cookie sheet.

Mix together the 2 Tbsp. buttermilk and 1 Tbsp. brown sugar and gently wash the tops of the scones. Place in the oven and bake for about 15 - 18 minutes until the tops of the scones are golden.

The refrigerator light goes on...

Baking requires precision and care should be taken if making substitutions. This is because baking is essentially chemistry. There is more latitude with cooking, but when working with lower calorie recipes, sometimes even subtle changes can ruin a recipe.

Nutrition Facts	
Serving size	1 scone
Servings	8
Calories 188	Calories from Fat 30
	% Daily Value
Total Fat 3 g	5 %
Saturated Fat 2 g	10 %
Trans Fat 0 g	
Monounsaturated Fat 1 g	
Cholesterol 9 mg	3 %
Sodium 297 mg	12 %
Total Carbohydrates 35 g	12 %
Dietary Fiber 1 g	4 %
Sugars 10 g	
Protein 4 g	
Vitamin A 2 %	Vitamin C 5 %
Calcium 11 %	Iron 10 %
Vitamin K 1 mcg	
Potassium 123 mg	
Magnesium 14 mg	

Pumpkin Nut Muffins

Servings: 6 | Serving size: 1 muffin

Cooking time: 30 minutes

This recipe can be multiplied by 2. Muffins will keep for 24 hours in a plastic bag. To freeze muffins, wrap individually. Remove from bag for 20 minutes to thaw. Slice in half and reheat in an oven that has been preheated to 300°F.

1 large	egg (separated)
2 tsp.	canola oil
1/2 cup	canned pumpkin
1/2 tsp.	pure vanilla extract
1/2 cup	Z-Sweet stevia or Splenda
1/4 cup	dried pumpkin seeds
2 Tbsp.	golden seedless raisins
1 cup	all purpose white flour
1/2 cup	whole wheat flour
2 Tbsp.	wheat germ
1/4 tsp.	salt
1 tsp.	baking powder
1/4 tsp.	baking soda
1/2 tsp.	ground nutmeg
1 tsp.	ground cinnamon
1/2 tsp.	ground allspice
1/3 cup	non-fat buttermilk
2 tsp.	light brown sugar

Preheat oven to 375°F.

Using a whisk, cream together the egg yolk and canola oil. Add the pumpkin and whisk into the mixture until well blended. Add the vanilla extract and Z-Sweet or Splenda and blend. Fold in the pumpkin seeds and raisins.

Sift the all purpose flour, whole wheat flour, wheat germ, salt, baking powder, baking soda, nutmeg, cinnamon, and allspice in a sifter and sift into the mixing bowl.

Gently fold the creamed mixture together with the flour mixture until smooth. When blended the mixture will still be dry. Whisk the egg white until it is white and foamy (about tripled in volume). Fold in the egg white.

Fold in the buttermilk and when the dough is just blended together stop.

Line a muffin tin with muffin papers and fill each muffin paper with an equal amount of batter. Sprinkle the brown sugar over the tops of the muffins. and then place the muffins in the oven and bake for 20 minutes.

The refrigerator light goes on...
Make muffins on a weekend day for a grab and go healthy breakfast. These are simple to make, keep well for a few days, and are not only delicious but have lots of fiber.

Nutrition Facts	
Serving size	1 muffin
Servings	12
Calories 225	Calories from Fat 61
	% Daily Value
Total Fat 7 g	11 %
Saturated Fat 1 g	7 %
Trans Fat 0 g	
Monounsaturated Fat 3 g	
Cholesterol 35 mg	12 %
Sodium 306 mg	13 %
Total Carbohydrates 33 g	11 %
Dietary Fiber 3 g	14 %
Sugars 5 g	
Protein 9 g	
Vitamin A 65 %	Vitamin C 2 %
Calcium 9 %	Iron 19 %
Vitamin K 9 mcg	
Potassium 268 mg	
Magnesium 84 mg	

Omelet

Servings: 2 | Serving size: 1/2 omelet

Cooking time: 30 minutes

This recipe is not easily multiplied. I do occasionally keep the other half of an omelet and make sandwiches with it.

1 tsp.	unsalted butter
1/3	bell pepper (julienne strips)
4	large egg whites
2	large egg yolks
1/8 tsp.	salt
3 Tbsp.	water
6	large fresh basil leaves (chiffonade)
	fresh ground black pepper
1/2 ounce	Parmigiano-Reggiano (grated)

Melt the butter in a small non-stick skillet pan over medium heat. Add the peppers and cook until they are browned but not limp. Remove and set aside.

In a small mixing bowl whisk together the egg whites, eggs yolks, salt and water. Add ground pepper to taste.

Heat a medium sized non-stick skillet over medium-high heat and place the basil in the bottom and pour the egg mixture over the top. Reduce the heat to medium heat and cook slowly. Gently slide a spatula under the eggs and carefully fold back the cooked portion so as to expose more uncooked egg to the bottom of the pan.

When the eggs are nearly set, add the peppers to the center (in a straight line so as to make folding easier). Fold the omelet in half over the peppers. Cook about 2 more minutes and remove.

Sprinkle the Parmigiano-Reggiano and the basil over the top of the omelet and then divide into two portions.

Serve.

The refrigerator light goes on...
Don't read nutrition facts looking for the perfect 30% of calories from fat or so many grams of carbohydrates. It is what you eat in a day and not one particular dish that's important.

Nutrition Facts	
Serving size	1/2 omelet
Servings	2
Calories 144	Calories from Fat 77
	% Daily Value
Total Fat 9 g	13 %
Saturated Fat 4 g	20 %
Trans Fat 0 g	
Monounsaturated Fat 3 g	
Cholesterol 220 mg	73 %
Sodium 383 mg	16 %
Total Carbohydrates 3 g	1 %
Dietary Fiber 1 g	4 %
Sugars 1 g	
Protein 13 g	
Vitamin A 29 %	Vitamin C 27 %
Calcium 11 %	Iron 4 %
Vitamin K 9 mcg	
Potassium 260 mg	
Magnesium 29 mg	

Apple Cinnamon Bread

Servings: 8 | Serving size: 1 slice

Cooking time: 75 minutes

This recipe can be multiplied by 2. Bread will keep for 72 - 96 hours in a plastic bag. Reheat gently. This will freeze fairly well if sealed tightly in a plastic bag.

1/4 cup	pecans (coarsely chopped)
2 tsp.	maple syrup
1/4 tsp.	ground cinnamon
1	large egg yolk
1 tsp.	canola oil
2/3 cup	Z-sweet stevia or Splenda
1/2 cup	unsweetened applesauce
1/2 tsp.	pure vanilla extract
3	large egg whites
1 1/4 cup	all purpose flour
3/4 cup	whole wheat flour
1/4 tsp.	salt
2 tsp.	baking powder
1/2 tsp.	baking soda
1 tsp.	ground cinnamon
1/4 cup	wheat germ
2 cups	apples (peeled and grated)
1/2 cup	non-fat buttermilk

Preheat oven to 350°F. Line a 1 1/2 quart glass Pyrex oblong loaf pan with foil (non-stick foil works best).

Combine the pecans, maple syrup and cinnamon in a small bowl. Stir until well blended. Set aside.

Whisk the egg yolk until smooth. Add the canola oil and whisk together until smooth. Add the Z-Sweet or Splenda, applesauce, and vanilla extract and whisk until smooth.

In separate bowl whisk the egg whites until they begin to be very frothy and white. Do not beat into stiff peaks.

Place the all-purpose flour, whole wheat flour, salt, baking powder, baking soda, cinnamon, and wheat germ in a sifter and sift into the mixing bowl.

Gently fold the creamed mixture together with the flour mixture. As this is blended add the grated apples.

Just as the apples are blended in, add the buttermilk and fold until smooth. As soon as the mixture is well blended, add the frothed egg whites and fold together until smooth.

Pour the batter into the lined Pyrex dish. Spread the pecan and maple syrup mixture evenly over the top and place in the preheated oven. Bake for 60 minutes.

The refrigerator light goes on...
Making bread is a little more difficult to make than a simple muffin recipe. This Apple Cinnamon quick bread is a great comfort food. Warm and inviting with the spicy cinnamon aroma, just having this one in the oven makes the house more homey. The loaf will keep well for about 3 - 4 days and it's best to cut two thin slices and toast them lightly in the oven or toaster oven.

Nutrition Facts	
Serving size	1 slice
Servings	8
Calories 196	Calories from Fat 39
	% Daily Value
Total Fat 5 g	7 %
Saturated Fat 1 g	3 %
Trans Fat 0 g	
Monounsaturated Fat 2 g	
Cholesterol 27 mg	9 %
Sodium 308 mg	13 %
Total Carbohydrates 33 g	11 %
Dietary Fiber 3 g	14 %
Sugars 6 g	
Protein 7 g	
Vitamin A 1 %	Vitamin C 2 %
Calcium 11 %	Iron 11 %
Vitamin K 1 mcg	
Potassium 200 mg	
Magnesium 37 mg	

Curried Chicken Salad

Servings: 3 as a dinner entrée, 6 for lunch | Serving size: about 3/4 cup

Cooking time: 30 minutes (does not include chilling time)

This recipe can be multiplied by 2. This recipe keeps well for about 24 - 36 hours only. Serve with one 6 inch whole wheat pita round and garnish with cucumbers or alfalfa sprouts.

4 cups	water
4 ounce	boneless, skinless chicken breasts
1 tsp.	curry powder
2 Tbsp.	reduced-fat mayonnaise
1 Tbsp.	slivered almonds
2 Tbsp.	non-fat sour cream
1/8 tsp.	cinnamon
1 Tbsp.	chutney
2 Tbsp.	golden raisins
2 Tbsp.	green onions (chopped)
1/4 cup	celery (diced)
1 Tbsp.	red bell pepper (diced)

Place water in a shallow pan over high heat. When the liquid is at a shiver, reduce the heat to medium so that it won't boil. Add the chicken breasts and poach until just done. This should take about 10 minutes; check for an internal temperature of 170° to ensure the chicken is cooked.

When the chicken is cooked, remove it to a cutting board and let it cool for about 15 minutes; then put it in the refrigerator to chill.

When chilled, cube the chicken breasts and place in a medium mixing bowl. Add all the other ingredients and fold together until well coated.

Chill for at least an hour before serving.

The refrigerator light goes on...
There are hundreds of ways to make chicken salad (or shrimp or tuna or etc.). Don't be timid. Mixing strong flavors, such as chutney, curry and raisins, makes for a rich taste while using less fat and calories.

Nutrition Facts	
Serving size	3/4 cup
Servings	3
Calories 141	Calories from Fat 46
	% Daily Value
Total Fat 5 g	8 %
Saturated Fat 1 g	4 %
Trans Fat 0 g	
Monounsaturated Fat 1 g	
Cholesterol 26 mg	9 %
Sodium 122 mg	5 %
Total Carbohydrates 14 g	5 %
Dietary Fiber 1 g	4 %
Sugars 9 g	
Protein 10 g	
Vitamin A 6 %	Vitamin C 11 %
Calcium 4 %	Iron 5 %
Vitamin K 27 mcg	
Potassium 244 mg	
Magnesium 23 mg	

Lentil and Black Bean Salad

Servings: 3 | Serving size: about 1 1/2 cups

Cooking time: 45 minutes (does not include chilling time)

This recipe can easily be multiplied by 2. This salad keeps well for 3 – 4 days and is better the second day.

1/2 cup	red lentils
1/2 cup	green lentils
6 cups	water (divided)
1 – 15 ounce can	black beans (drained and rinsed)
1 large	shallot (minced)
1 rib	celery (sliced thin)
1/4 tsp.	red pepper flakes
1 Tbsp.	extra virgin olive oil
2 Tbsp.	white wine vinegar
1 Tbsp.	maple syrup
1/4 tsp.	salt
to taste	fresh ground black pepper

Cook the red lentils in 3 cups of simmering water for about 15 – 20 minutes, until just tender. Drain and rinse with cold water.

Cook the green lentils in 3 cups of simmering water for about 15 – 20 minutes, until just tender. Drain and rinse with cold water.

Combine the green and red lentils with the black beans.

Add the shallot, celery, red bell pepper, olive oil, vinegar, maple syrup, salt and pepper.

Chill overnight.

The refrigerator light goes on...
Lentils are amazingly high in fiber and taste great.

Nutrition Facts	
Serving size	1 1/2 cup
Servings	3
Calories 514	Calories from Fat 54
	% Daily Value
Total Fat 6 g	10 %
Saturated Fat 1 g	5 %
Trans Fat 0 g	
Monounsaturated Fat 4 g	
Cholesterol 0 mg	0 %
Sodium 220 mg	9 %
Total Carbohydrates 85 g	28 %
Dietary Fiber 30 g	119 %
Sugars 7 g	
Protein 31 g	
Vitamin A 7 %	Vitamin C 10 %
Calcium 3 %	Iron 47 %
Vitamin K 17 mcg	
Potassium 1677 mg	
Magnesium 195 mg	

Thai Cucumber Salad

Servings: 4 | Serving size: about 1 cup salad as a side dish

Cooking time: 30 minutes (does not include chilling or marinating time)

This recipe can easily be multiplied by 2 or 3. Leftovers are good for 24 hours at the most.

1 cup	rice vinegar
1 tsp	lime zest
1/4 tsp.	Tabasco sauce
2 Tbsp.	Z-sweet stevia or Splenda
1/2 cup	red onion (diced)
2 large	cucumbers (peeled and sliced thin)
1/4 cup	cilantro leaves
1 Tbsp.	raw peanuts (chopped)

Combine the rice vinegar, lime zest, Tabasco, Splenda or stevia, red onion, cucumber slices and cilantro leaves in a glass or stainless steel bowl.

You can add the peanuts now and let them marinate. They will be slightly chewy. I prefer to sprinkle them over the top of the salad when I am serving.

Marinate at least 2 hours.

The refrigerator light goes on...
When I was a kid in Atlanta my mom used to make cucumbers and onions with white vinegar, a touch of salt and pepper and just enough sugar to take the bite off. The flavors are the same – Southeast America, Southeast Asia – just subtle differences.

Nutrition Facts	
Serving size	1 cup salad
Servings	4
Calories 46	Calories from Fat 11
	% Daily Value
Total Fat 1 g	2 %
Saturated Fat <1 g	1 %
Trans Fat 0 g	
Monounsaturated Fat 0 g	
Cholesterol 0 mg	0 %
Sodium 8 mg	0 %
Total Carbohydrates 5 g	2 %
Dietary Fiber 1 g	5 %
Sugars 3 g	
Protein 1 g	
Vitamin A 3 %	Vitamin C 10 %
Calcium 3 %	Iron 3 %
Vitamin K 10 mcg	
Potassium 229 mg	
Magnesium 21 mg	

Mediterranean Chicken Salad

Servings: 4 | Serving size: about 2 cups salad

Cooking time: 45 minutes

This recipe can easily be multiplied by 2. It makes great leftovers and is actually better the second day. Keep in refrigerator for no more than 48 hours.

1 clove	garlic (minced)
1 lb.	boneless skinless chicken breasts (sliced into thin strips)
	spray olive oil
1 large	red onion (sliced)
1/2	red bell pepper (sliced into thin strips)
1/2	yellow bell pepper (sliced into thin strips)
1 small	zucchini (cut into large dice)
8 oz.	grape tomatoes
1 Tbsp.	extra virgin olive oil
2 Tbsp.	balsamic vinegar
1 Tbsp.	honey
1/2 tsp.	salt
to taste	fresh ground black pepper
12	black olives (cut in quarters)
8 leaves	fresh basil (chiffonade)
8 leaves	romaine lettuce
1 - 2 oz.	whole wheat roll (per serving)
1/2 oz.	goat cheese (per serving)

Preheat oven to 350°F. Place a large non-stick grill pan and a large non-stick skillet in the oven. (Two large non-stick skillets will do.).

While the oven is heating combine the minced garlic and chicken breast strips in a bowl and place the bowl in the refrigerator.

When the pans are hot spray each lightly with olive oil and add the sliced red onion to the grill pan and the zucchini and grape tomatoes to the skillet. Cook the tomatoes and zucchini for about 5 to 7 minutes tossing twice to make sure that they are well seared. Remove before the tomatoes get soft and place in a large bowl to cool in the refrigerator. Return the skillet to the oven.

Cook the onions tossing frequently until they begin to brown. Add the red and yellow pepper strips and cook for about 5 to 7 minutes tossing once or twice. Remove before the peppers get too soft and add to the cooling tomato/zucchini mixture and toss well.

Spray the large skillet lightly again with olive oil and add the garlic and chicken strips. Cook for about 10 minutes tossing once or twice. Make sure the chicken is cooked through. Remove and add to the roasted vegetable mixture tossing to coat well.

Add the olive oil, balsamic vinegar, honey, salt, pepper, olives and basil. Toss to coat the salad well and then return to the refrigerator to chill for at least 2 hours. When ready to serve, cut the romaine lettuce into strips and fold into the salad.

Slice the rolls and then heat gently. Serve spread with goat cheese.

Nutrition Facts	
Serving size	2 cups w/rolls and goat cheese
Servings	4
Calories 422	Calories from Fat 109
	% Daily Value
Total Fat 12 g	4 %
Saturated Fat 4 g	1 %
Trans Fat 0 g	
Monounsaturated Fat 0 g	
Cholesterol 0 mg	0 %
Sodium 149 mg	6 %
Total Carbohydrates 9 g	3 %
Dietary Fiber 4 g	16 %
Sugars 3 g	
Protein 1 g	
Vitamin A 1 %	Vitamin C 33 %
Calcium 1 %	Iron 3 %
Vitamin K 2 mcg	
Potassium 143 mg	
Magnesium 12 mg	

Zucchini Salad

Servings: 4 | Serving size: about 1 1/2 cup salad

Cooking time: 30 minutes (does not include chilling time)

This recipe can easily be halved or multiplied and keeps well for 2 - 3 days in the refrigerator.

2 Tbsp	olive oil
2 Tbsp	balsamic vinegar
2 Tbsp	maple syrup
1/4 tsp	salt
to taste	fresh ground black pepper
1 tsp	dried marjoram
1 lb	zucchini (cut into medium dice)
8 ounces	grape or cherry tomatoes
4 Tbsp	pine nuts

Whisk together the olive oil, balsamic vinegar, maple syrup, salt, pepper and marjoram. Place in the refrigerator while cutting the zucchini.

Cut the zucchini into medium dice. This should be about 1/4 inch cubes.

Toss the zucchini, tomatoes and pine nuts together in the vinaigrette. Chill well before serving.

The refrigerator light goes on...
This little salad is quick and easy and really tasty. You can use yellow squash instead or combine the two for great color. It makes a great side dish for almost any soup and then you have the perfect dinner.

Nutrition Facts	
Serving size	about 1 1/2 cup salad
Servings	4
Calories 180	Calories from Fat 117
	% Daily Value
Total Fat 13 g	17 %
Saturated Fat 1.5 g	7 %
Trans Fat 0 g	
Monounsaturated Fat 7 g	
Cholesterol 0 mg	0 %
Sodium 160 mg	7 %
Total Carbohydrates 15 g	5 %
Dietary Fiber 2 g	8 %
Sugars 12 g	
Protein 3 g	
Vitamin A 4 %	Vitamin C 31 %
Calcium 3 %	Iron 7 %
Vitamin K 20 mcg	
Potassium 500 mg	

Spaghetti Squash Salad

Servings: 8 | Serving size = about one cup

Cooking time: 30 minutes (does not include chilling time)

This recipe can easily be halved. This recipe keeps well for up to 3 days.

2 quarts	water
1	spaghetti squash
3 Tbsp.	olive oil
4 tsp.	balsamic vinegar
1 Tbsp.	pure maple syrup
1 medium	red bell pepper (diced)
1 large	shallot (minced)
1/2 tsp.	salt
to taste	fresh ground black pepper

Place the water in a large stock pot over high heat.

When the water is boiling add the spaghetti squash and reduce the heat to a slow boil. Cook for 25 minutes and remove from the water. Let the squash rest on the counter to cool.

Cut the cooled squash open lengthwise and remove the seeds. Scoop out the flesh of the squash gently dividing the strands.

Toss the squash with the olive oil, vinegar, maple syrup, red pepper, shallot, salt and pepper. Chill well.

The refrigerator light goes on...
This is a perfect lunch salad. Pair this with a hearty whole grain roll lightly toasted and smeared with just a bit of cheese and you can taste the summer any time of year.

Nutrition Facts	
Serving size	1 cup
Servings	4
Calories 118	Calories from Fat 51
	% Daily Value
Total Fat 6 g	9 %
Saturated Fat 1 g	4 %
Trans Fat 0 g	
Monounsaturated Fat 4 g	
Cholesterol 0 mg	0 %
Sodium 164 mg	7 %
Total Carbohydrates 17 g	6 %
Dietary Fiber 1 g	4 %
Sugars 5 g	
Protein 2 g	
Vitamin A 32 %	Vitamin C 96 %
Calcium 4 %	Iron 5 %
Vitamin K 5 mcg	
Potassium 289 mg	
Magnesium 24 mg	

Roasted Eggplant Salad

Servings: 8 | Serving size: about one cup

Cooking time: 60 minutes

This recipe can easily be multiplied by 2 or halved. This recipe keeps well in the refrigerator for about 72 hours.

	spray olive oil
2 lbs.	eggplant (cut into 1/2 inch cubes)
2 medium	yellow onions (cut into 1/8th wedges)
1 pint	grape tomatoes
1/4 cup	slivered almonds
1/2 tsp.	salt
to taste	fresh ground black pepper
2 Tbsp.	extra virgin olive oil
3 Tbsp.	balsamic vinegar
1/4 cup	fresh basil (chiffonade)
1 Tbsp.	fresh oregano
1 bulb	roasted garlic (chopped)

Preheat oven to 325°F. Place a large roasting pan in the oven. When the oven is hot lightly spray the pan with oil and add the eggplant, onions, tomatoes and almonds.

Return the pan to the oven and roast for about 30 - 40 minutes. Stir the vegetables about every 10 minutes. They may require a light spray once or twice with the oil to keep them from sticking.

Remove form the oven and let the vegetables cool slightly. Place in a large mixing bowl and add the salt, pepper, olive oil, vinegar, basil, oregano and roasted garlic.

Stir well and chill.

** The garlic can be roasted at the same time as the vegetables using the Roasted Garlic recipe. Alternatively, add 5 cloves of minced garlic with the veggies before roasting. The flavor will be less subtle but is quite good (and the recipe is easier if you haven't roasted the garlic).

The refrigerator light goes on...

This is a very easy recipe and the salad goes with everything. You can serve it under fish or with a pasta recipe as a side dish. It's great to take to a pot luck and everyone will love you for it (and they don't even have to know that it's healthy).

Nutrition Facts	
Serving size	1 cup
Servings	4
Calories 118	Calories from Fat 58
	% Daily Value
Total Fat 7 g	10 %
Saturated Fat 1 g	4 %
Trans Fat 0 g	
Monounsaturated Fat 4 g	
Cholesterol 0 mg	0 %
Sodium 151 mg	6 %
Total Carbohydrates 14 g	5 %
Dietary Fiber 5 g	22 %
Sugars 5 g	
Protein 3 g	
Vitamin A 7 %	Vitamin C 16 %
Calcium 5 %	Iron 5 %
Vitamin K 14 mcg	
Potassium 445 mg	
Magnesium 41 mg	

Black Eyed Pea Salad

Servings: 4 | Serving size: about one cup

Cooking time: 90 minutes

This recipe can easily be multiplied by 2 or 3. This recipe is better if made the night before and it keeps well for about 48 hours in the fridge.

3 quarts	water
2 1/3 cups	dried black eyed peas
1 medium	carrot (peeled and diced)
1 rib	celery (diced)
2 Tbsp.	red onion (minced)
1/3	green bell pepper (seeded and diced)
1 Tbsp.	grapeseed oil
1 Tbsp.	pure maple syrup
2 Tbsp.	apple cider vinegar
1/2 tsp.	salt
1/8 tsp.	fresh ground black pepper
2 Tbsp.	fresh dill (chopped)

Rinse the peas well and place in a large pot. Cover with cold water and soak overnight if possible. Drain the peas and replace with 3 quarts of cold water. Cook the peas for about an hour.

** An alternative, quicker method is to place the peas in a pot and cover with cold water. Bring to a boil and cook for two minutes. Remove the peas from the heat rinse and lest stand one hour. Rinse and place in a pot with 3 quarts of cold water. Cook the peas for about an hour until soft.

** Canned no salt added black eyed peas may be used. Rinse well. You will need two 15 ounce cans for this recipe.

When the beans are cooked, drain well and cool. Place in a medium mixing bowl and add the carrot, celery, bell pepper, grapeseed oil, maple syrup, vinegar, salt, pepper and fresh dill. Toss well and chill at least an hour.

The refrigerator light goes on...
You wouldn't think that black eyed peas are all that good for you but they are. The cheap, lowly black eye is a member of the legume family and chock full of everything good for you. A great ingredient as a side dish with your Oven Fried Chicken or used in a salad.

Nutrition Facts	
Serving size	1 cup
Servings	4
Calories 208	Calories from Fat 36
	% Daily Value
Total Fat 4 g	6 %
Saturated Fat 1 g	3 %
Trans Fat 0 g	
Monounsaturated Fat 1 g	
Cholesterol 0 mg	0 %
Sodium 320 mg	13 %
Total Carbohydrates 33 g	11 %
Dietary Fiber 9 g	38 %
Sugars 9 g	
Protein 10 g	
Vitamin A 55 %	Vitamin C 24 %
Calcium 5 %	Iron 19 %
Vitamin K 10 mcg	
Potassium 499 mg	
Magnesium 75 mg	

Pizza with Tomato, Basil and Roasted Garlic

Servings: 3 | Serving size: 1 individual pizza

Cooking time: 30 minutes

This recipe can easily be multiplied by 2, 3 or 4. Leftovers are good cold for breakfast. This recipe requires Whole Wheat Pizza Dough and Roasted Garlic to be made first (recipes included).

1 medium (4 ounce)	tomato
1 ounce	fresh mozzarella
8 large	fresh basil leaves
4 cloves	roasted garlic
1/2 ounce	Parmigiano-Reggiano (grated)
1/4	whole wheat pizza dough

Preheat the oven to 500°F.

Pizza is best baked on a pizza stone but a cookie sheet will work as well. Place the baking stone or cookie sheet in the oven and allow it to heat at least 15 - 20 minutes.

While the baking surface is heating, slice tomato in half vertically. Remove the seeds and slice the tomato into julienne strips.

Cut the fresh mozzarella into 1/2 inch cubes.

Gently slice the basil into strips.

Cut each clove of roasted garlic into quarters.

Gently toss the tomato strips, mozzarella, basil leaves and garlic together in a small mixing bowl.

Set the tomato mixture close to the oven so that it will be accessible and easy to place on top of the dough. Have the grated parmesan within easy reach.

Using 1/4 of the pizza dough recipe (for each pizza) gently stretch into 8-inch rounds. Don't work too hard to get a perfectly round shape.

Once the dough is formed, place it on the hot pizza stone and top with the tomato/mozzarella mix-ture.

Bake for approximately eight minutes, and then top with the Parmesan cheese. Bake for another 3 – 5 minutes - until the cheese has melted. Remove from the oven and let it cool for about 90 seconds, slice and serve.

The refrigerator light goes on...
A pizza stone is the key to baking a professional quality pie. They are inexpensive and so worth using.

Nutrition Facts		
Serving size	1 pizza (includes dough and toppings)	
Servings		1
Calories 479	Calories from Fat 109	
		% Daily Value
Total Fat 12 g		19 %
Saturated Fat 6 g		32 %
Trans Fat 0 g		
Monounsaturated Fat 4 g		
Cholesterol 32 mg		11 %
Sodium 708 mg		30 %
Total Carbohydrates 73 g		24 %
Dietary Fiber 10 g		40 %
Sugars 11 g		
Protein 24 g		
Vitamin A 13 %	Vitamin C 35 %	
Calcium 41 %	Iron 31 %	
Vitamin K 24 mcg		
Potassium 713 mg		
Magnesium 125 mg		

Whole Wheat Pizza Dough

Servings: enough dough for 4 individual pizzas
Serving size: 1 individual pizza

Cooking time: 90 minutes

This recipe is easily multiplied by 2 or cut in half. This dough will keep for about 36 hours in the refrigerator if wrapped tightly in plastic wrap. It will not be as good as fresh.

1 cup	warm water
1 tsp.	dry active yeast
4 tsp.	honey
2 cups	whole wheat flour (does not need to be sifted)
1/2 cup	all purpose flour (does not need to be sifted)
1/2 tsp.	salt

Heat the water in the microwave until warm to touch – about 110°F to 115°F. (I prefer to use a thermometer for this because if the water is too hot you will kill the yeast.)

Place the yeast and honey in a large mixing bowl and pour the heated water over the mixture, stirring until well blended. Let the mixture stand for about 5 - 7 minutes until foamy.

Add the whole wheat flour, all purpose flour and salt and stir with a fork until a coarse dough forms.

Continue to mix by hand until a dough ball forms and all the flour is well blended.

Cover the bowl and place it in a sink with about 4 inches of hot water in the bottom. The heat from the warm water will help the dough rise. The dough will double in size in about 30 – 40 minutes. Punch it a few times with your fingers and let it rise another 30 minutes.

Remove from the bowl and cut the ball into four equal pieces. Cover the dough that you are not going to use immediately in plastic wrap and chill.

The refrigerator light goes on...
Using whole wheat pizza dough for pizza recipes is a great way to get extra fiber. The dough has more body than regular pizza dough and a mellow, sweet flavor. And it adds 6 grams of fiber to your diet!

Nutrition Facts	
Serving size	1 pizza
Servings	4
Calories 284	Calories from Fat 9
	% Daily Value
Total Fat 1 g	5 %
Saturated Fat 0 g	0 %
Trans Fat 0 g	
Monounsaturated Fat 0 g	
Cholesterol 0 mg	0 %
Sodium 295 mg	12 %
Total Carbohydrates 61 g	20 %
Dietary Fiber 8 g	32 %
Sugars 6 g	
Protein 10 g	
Vitamin A 0 %	Vitamin C 0 %
Calcium 2 %	Iron 18 %
Vitamin K 1 mcg	
Potassium 283 mg	
Magnesium 87 mg	

Roasted Garlic

Servings: 6 | Serving Size: 1/3 head of garlic (about 6 cloves)

Cooking time: 60 minutes

I make up to about 4 heads of garlic at a time. This keeps well, tightly covered, for about 4 - 6 days.

2 heads	whole garlic
2 tsp.	extra virgin olive oil

Preheat oven to 300°F.

Peel the outermost skin of the garlic only. With the bulb whole, turn on its side and slice 1/2-inch of the stem end off the garlic bulbs.

Pour the olive oil in the bottom of a heavy bottom sauce pan.

Place the garlic cut side down in the pan.

Cover and roast for 45 minutes until cloves are slightly brown at the cut end and soft throughout.

The refrigerator light goes on...
Roasted garlic is a staple in my kitchen and should be in yours. I generally roast about 3 heads every ten days or so. It makes a great ingredient in mashed potatoes and also enriches any sauce. It is fantastic served as hors d'oeuvres on bread with some soft goat cheese and veggies.

Nutrition Facts		
Serving size	1/3 head of garlic (about 4 cloves)	
Servings		6
Calories 40	Calories from Fat 14	
		% Daily Value
Total Fat 2 g		2 %
Saturated Fat 0 g		1 %
Trans Fat 0 g		
Monounsaturated Fat 0 g		
Cholesterol 0 mg		0 %
Sodium 3 mg		0 %
Total Carbohydrates 6 g		2 %
Dietary Fiber 0 g		2 %
Sugars 0 g		
Protein 1 g		
Vitamin A 0 %	Vitamin C 9 %	
Calcium 3 %	Iron 2 %	
Vitamin K 1 mcg		
Potassium 72 mg		
Magnesium 5 mg		

Butternut Squash Risotto

Servings: 4 | Serving size: about 2 cups

Cooking time: 45 minutes

This recipe can easily be multiplied by 2. Leftovers are good. Reheat gently.

2 lbs	butternut squash
	spray olive oil
2 tsp	extra virgin olive oil
1 large	leek
1/2 medium	red onion (diced)
1 cup	arborio rice
3 cups	water
1 cup	low sodium chicken or vegetable broth
1/4 cup	dry sherry
1/4 tsp	salt
to taste	fresh ground black pepper
1/4 tsp	ground paprika
1 1/2 ounces	Parmigiano-Reggiano (grated)

Preheat the oven to 325°F.

Slice the squash lengthwise and remove the seeds. Spray lightly with olive oil and place in the pre-heated oven, cut side up. Roast the squash for about 1 hour, until slightly tender.

Remove from the oven and let cool. The squash will have a small amount of liquid in the cavity. After it is cool, drain the liquid and place the squash on a cutting board, cut side down.

Gently peel the skin away from the squash. Slice across the squash parallel to the cutting board, dividing into three slices. Keep the shape of the squash intact. Slice lengthwise at about 1/4 inch intervals and then crosswise, so as to divide into 1/2 inch cubes. Set aside.

Slice the root off of the leek. Slice the leek in half, separating the white from the green tops. Clean the green tops under running water and slice very thin. Slice the white part of the leek very thin lengthwise and clean well.

Heat the olive oil in a large sauce pan over high heat and add the green part of the leek. Reduce the heat to medium-high and cook very slowly. Stir frequently.

When the leek is wilted, add the white part of the leek and the diced red onion. Reduce the heat to medium and cook for about five minutes, until the onions begin to soften.

Place the rice in the pan with the onions and leeks and stir for about 3 minutes. Add two cups of water, the chicken stock, sherry, salt and pepper. Cook over medium-high heat stirring frequently. Add the remaining water, 1 cup at a time.

Add the ground paprika and continue cooking. The rice will take about 20 to 25 minutes to cook and may require more water be added. Stir frequently, using about 1/2 cup of water at a time as needed, until the rice is soft but not mushy and there is a small amount of creamy sauce.

Stir in the Parmigiano-Reggiano until it is melted and then gently fold in the diced butternut squash. Serve.

Nutrition Facts	
Serving size	About 2 cups risotto
Servings	4
Calories 390	Calories from Fat 63
	% Daily Value
Total Fat 7 g	8 %
Saturated Fat 2 g	10 %
Trans Fat 0 g	
Monounsaturated Fat 2.5 g	
Cholesterol 10 mg	3 %
Sodium 360 mg	15 %
Total Carbohydrates 72 g	26 %
Dietary Fiber 7 g	26 %
Sugars 10 g	
Protein 13 g	
Vitamin A 140 %	Vitamin C 59 %
Calcium 17 %	Iron 12 %
Vitamin K 10 mcg	
Potassium 900 mg	

Seared Tuna Steak with Sake-Wasabi Sauce

Servings: 2 | Serving size = 4 ounce tuna steak

Cooking time: 30 minutes

This recipe can easily be multiplied by 2 but re-quires two large pans. Leftover tuna makes great tuna sandwiches or salads. Serve with Brown Rice (recipe included).

2 tsp.	low-sodium soy sauce
1 Tbsp.	sake
1 Tbsp.	fresh lime juice
2 Tbsp.	honey
1 tsp.	wasabi paste
2 - 4 ounce	tuna steaks (about 1 1/2 inch thick)
1/8 tsp.	salt
	fresh ground black pepper
1 tsp.	dark sesame oil

Mix the soy sauce, sake, lime juice, honey and wasabi paste together in a small bowl. Whisk until the wasabi is completely dissolved. This can be done a day in advance and refrigerated.

Rinse the tuna steaks and pat dry. Sprinkle one side with the salt and then pepper liberally on that side.

Place the sake sauce in a small sauce pan and heat over low heat. Do not allow the sauce to boil.

Set the oven to warm and place serving plates inside.

Heat the sesame oil in a large non-stick skillet over high until very hot (almost smoking). Add the tuna steaks, seasoned side down. Cook over medium-high heat until well seared and turn. Rare tuna will take about 4 - 5 minutes per side.

Remove the plates from the oven and spoon about 4 tablespoons of the heated sauce into the bottom of each plate.

This dish is made to be served with Brown Rice (recipe included) but any rice will do. When the tuna is done mound a serving of rice in the center of the plate on top of the sauce and place the tuna on top. Garnish by sprinkling the chopped scallions over the fish and serve.

The refrigerator light goes on...
Searing any meat, such as tuna, makes for a rich and luxurious dish and is a healthy cooking technique. Make sure that the pan is very hot and add the meat carefully so as to not splash any hot oil.

Nutrition Facts	
Serving size	1 tuna steak
Servings	4
Calories 227	Calories from Fat 30
	% Daily Value
Total Fat 3 g	5 %
Saturated Fat 1 g	3 %
Trans Fat 0 g	
Monounsaturated Fat 1 g	
Cholesterol 51 mg	17 %
Sodium 372 mg	15 %
Total Carbohydrates 20 g	7 %
Dietary Fiber 1 g	3 %
Sugars 18 g	
Protein 27 g	
Vitamin A 4 %	Vitamin C 12 %
Calcium 4 %	Iron 7 %
Vitamin K 32 mcg	
Potassium 587 mg	
Magnesium 64 mg	

Linguine with Shrimp in Vodka Tomato Cream Sauce

Servings: 4 | Serving Size: 2 oz. pasta/4 oz. shrimp

Cooking time: 45 minutes

This recipe can easily be multiplied by 2 if you use a large skillet. Leftovers are fair at best. This recipe requires Tomato Sauce (recipe included) to be made first.

1 cup	water
1/2 cup	sun-dried tomatoes (sliced)
3 cups	water
16 spears	asparagus
4 tsp.	unsalted butter
1 lb.	large shrimp (peeled & deveined)
1 cup	shallots (sliced)
1/2 cup	vodka
1 cup	tomato sauce (recipe included)
1 cup	2% milk
1/4 tsp.	salt
5 quarts	water
8 ounces	linguine
2 Tbsp	fresh basil (chiffonade)

Heat 1 cup water until boiling and pour over the sun-dried tomatoes. Allow to stand for about 15 minutes, until soft and then drain the liquid into a sauce pan. Heat the liquid on high heat until it boils and reduce to 1/4 cup. Set aside.

Heat 3 cups of water to the shiver stage in a medium skillet. Add the asparagus and blanch for about 2 - 3 minutes, until they just begin to turn bright green. Remove and let dry on a paper towel. When they are cool, cut them in 2 inch segments.

Melt the butter in a large skillet over medium-high heat. Add the shrimp and sauté until slightly firm (no more than about 2 minutes on each side). Remove shrimp to a plate.

Begin heating the 5 quarts of water in a large pot. Add the linguine and cook about 15 minutes until just done (the pasta should have a slightly firm texture).

As the pasta is cooking, add the shallots to the skillet and cook over medium heat until they begin to soften and turn slightly brown (about 7 - 10 minutes).

Reduce the heat to low, add the vodka and cook briefly; then add the reduced water from the sun dried tomatoes, tomato sauce, milk and salt. After this has cooked for about 3 minutes, add the asparagus and sun-dried tomatoes. Simmer until tomatoes are tender (about 4 minutes). Add shrimp; toss to coat and allow to cook for another 4 minutes, until the shrimp is heated through.

Drain the linguine. Add the pasta to the tomato sauce and toss to coat well. Season to taste with fresh ground black pepper.

Served topped with basil.

The refrigerator light goes on...
519 calories may seem like a lot, but look carefully at the Nutrition Facts. This is a complete meal and it has so much going for it. It is low in fat and cholesterol, and has tomatoes, asparagus, tons of vitamins, and lycopenes -- all in one pasta bowl.

Nutrition Facts	
Serving size 2 oz. pasta/4 oz. shrimp	
Servings	4
Calories 519	Calories from Fat 72
	% Daily Value
Total Fat 8 g	13 %
Saturated Fat 4 g	19 %
Trans Fat 0 g	
Monounsaturated Fat 2 g	
Cholesterol 185 mg	62 %
Sodium 500 mg	21 %
Total Carbohydrates 60 g	22 %
Dietary Fiber 4 g	16 %
Sugars 9 g	
Protein 36 g	
Vitamin A 28 %	Vitamin C 22 %
Calcium 20 %	Iron 40 %
Vitamin K 36 mcg	
Potassium 954 mg	
Magnesium 113 mg	

Fettuccine with Dill Pesto and Shrimp

Servings: 2 | Serving size: 2 oz. pasta, 3 oz. shrimp

Cooking time: 30 minutes

This recipe requires Dill Pesto be made first (recipe included). This recipe will keep fairly well for a day or so.

4 ounces	whole wheat fettuccine
4 quarts	water
1 tsp.	extra virgin olive oil
6 ounces	fresh shrimp (peeled and deveined)
2 Tbsp.	dill pesto
1/4 cup	chicken stock
4 ounces	asparagus spears (steamed)
1/2 ounce	Parmigiano-Reggiano (grated)

Heat the water over high heat in a large stock-pot until boiling. Add the fettuccine.

Place the asparagus in a steamer and as the pasta nears being done (about ten minutes) turn the heat on high.

Heat the olive oil in a large non-stick skillet over medium-high heat.

Add the shrimp and cook on one side for about 2 minutes. Turn and reduce the heat to medium-low and cook for another two minutes.

Add the pesto and chicken stock and toss to coat the shrimp well.

Drain the pasta and add to the pan with the shrimp and pesto.

Divide the steamed asparagus between the two pasta bowls. Fill each bowl with 1/2 of the shrimp/pesto/fettuccini and divide the grated Parmigiano-Reggiano evenly over the top of each dish.

The refrigerator light goes on...
You're not stuck with using basil for your pesto. Almost any green, such as cilantro or arugula, will work.

Nutrition Facts		
Serving size		2 oz. pasta
Servings		2
Calories 404	Calories from Fat 95	
		% Daily Value
Total Fat 11 g		17 %
Saturated Fat 2 g		12 %
Trans Fat 0 g		
Monounsaturated Fat 4 g		
Cholesterol 134 mg		45 %
Sodium 249 mg		10 %
Total Carbohydrates 42 g		14 %
Dietary Fiber 3 g		11 %
Sugars 1 g		
Protein 33 g		
Vitamin A 17 %	Vitamin C 13 %	
Calcium 0 %	Iron 33 %	
Vitamin K 25 mcg		
Potassium 454 mg		
Magnesium 85 mg		

Meatloaf

Servings: 6 | Serving size: 1/6th meatloaf

Cooking time: 75 minutes

This keeps well for about 48 hours in the fridge after being cooked. This recipe requires that Tomato Sauce (recipe included) be made first.

1 lb.	extra lean ground beef
4 ounces	fresh bread crumbs
1 tsp.	dried oregano
1 tsp.	dried basil
1 tsp.	dried rosemary
1 tsp.	dried thyme
1/2 tsp.	salt
1/8 tsp.	fresh ground black pepper
3/4 cup	tomato sauce

Preheat oven to 325°F.

Line an oblong Pyrex dish or large skillet with aluminum foil.

Mix the ground beef together with the bread crumbs, oregano, basil, rosemary, thyme, salt and pepper until well blended.

Roll the mixture into a large ball and then shape into a loaf. Place the loaf in the aluminum foil lined pan. Continue to shape until the loaf is firm by pressing it together.

Place the pan in the oven. Cook for about 30 minutes and top with the marinara sauce. Return to the oven and cook for about 20 minutes until the internal temperature is 150°F. Remove from the oven and let rest for about 5 – 10 minutes before slicing.

The refrigerator light goes on...
Meatloaf, next to Mac and Cheese, may be the ultimate comfort food. It's great out of the oven and I like the tomato sauce topping. Served with mashed potatoes and a side of veggies and you can't help but feel good. As with all recipes that use ground beef, look for extra lean or 93 % lean. If need be, ask the butcher to grind you some from a piece of very well trimmed bottom round.

Bottled tomato sauce or marinara sauce will work well with this recipe. Look for a sauce with as little sodium as possible and 2 grams of fat or less per 1/2 cup serving.

Nutrition Facts	
Serving size	1 slice
Servings	6
Calories 193	Calories from Fat 44
	% Daily Value
Total Fat 5 g	8 %
Saturated Fat 2 g	10 %
Trans Fat 0 g	
Monounsaturated Fat 2 g	
Cholesterol 47 mg	16 %
Sodium 387 mg	16 %
Total Carbohydrates 17 g	6 %
Dietary Fiber 2 g	7 %
Sugars 0 g	
Protein 19 g	
Vitamin A 3 %	Vitamin C 8 %
Calcium 6 %	Iron 19 %
Vitamin K 8 mcg	
Potassium 425 mg	
Magnesium 33 mg	

Roasted Salmon with Red Thai Curry

Servings: 2 | Serving Size: 4 oz. salmon with sauce

Cooking time: 30 minutes

This recipe can be halved or multiplied by 2 or 3. Does not keep well but the sauce can be made up to 24 hours in advance. This recipe is great served over steamed napa cabbage but it's fantastic served over Plain Mashed Potatoes (recipe included).

1/2 tsp.	hot red bean paste
1/2 cup	light coconut milk
1 tsp.	lime zest
1 lime	juiced
1 tsp.	honey
2 Tbsp.	sake
2 tsp.	sesame oil
1/2 lb.	shiitake mushrooms (sliced)
2	4 oz. salmon filets
1 Tbsp.	low sodium soy sauce
2 Tbsp.	cilantro leaves

Place a large non-stick skillet in the oven and pre-heat to 450°F.

Mix together the red curry paste, coconut milk, lemon peel, Splenda, lime juice and sake. Whisk until smooth.

When the pan is hot, place the sesame oil in and swirl to coat the inside. Add the sliced shiitake mushrooms to the pan and return to the oven. Check every 3 minutes or so and shake the pan. After about 10 – 12 minutes the mushrooms will be a roasted brown.

Sprinkle the salt over the flesh side of the salmon. Place the filets in the hot pan flesh side down and return to the oven. Cook for about 4 minutes and turn the skin side down. Add the curry sauce and swirl. Return the pan to the oven and cook for another 4 – 5 minutes for rare. Remove and serve.

The refrigerator light goes on...
This is a really delicious recipe and one of those that you should be able to make from ingredients in your well stocked pantry.

Limes keep well, as do cans of coconut milk, sake (or even dry white wine), and hot red bean paste (or sambal or harissa - see below). If you keep these ingredients on hand, it will be easier and easier to cook and eat healthy.

While this recipe calls for red bean paste, you could use similar hot sauces in a pinch, such as sambal or harissa. The amount will depend on how hot the harissa or sambal is - I've had some that are very mild and some that could curl your eyelashes.

Nutrition Facts	
Serving size	4 oz. salmon w/sauce
Servings	2
Calories 370	Calories from Fat 207
	% Daily Value
Total Fat 23 g	30 %
Saturated Fat 7 g	34 %
Trans Fat 0 g	
Monounsaturated Fat 6 g	
Cholesterol 60 mg	32 %
Sodium 370 mg	16 %
Total Carbohydrates 11 g	4 %
Dietary Fiber 3 g	11 %
Sugars 3 g	
Protein 27 g	
Vitamin A 8 %	Vitamin C 11 %
Calcium 0 %	Iron 8 %
Vitamin K 5 mcg	
Potassium 900 mg	

Indian Shrimp Curry

Servings: 4 | Serving size: 4 oz. shrimp w/sauce

Cooking time: 30 minutes

This recipe can easily be multiplied by 2 or 3. Leftovers are great. Reheat gently. Serve over Jasmine Rice.

2 tsp.	extra virgin olive oil
2 cloves	garlic (minced)
1 medium	white onion (sliced)
1 medium	red onion (sliced)
1 cup	2% milk (divided)
1 Tbsp.	corn starch
1 Tbsp.	curry powder
2 tsp.	garam masala
2 tsp.	honey
1/2 tsp.	salt
1 cup	low-fat (lite) unsweetened coconut milk
1 lb.	large shrimp (peeled and deveined)
4 Tbsp.	fresh cilantro leaves

Heat the olive oil in large non-stick skillet over medium-high heat.

Add the garlic and onion and reduce the heat to medium.

Cook gently, stirring frequently, until the onions begin to soften.

While the onions are cooking, place the cornstarch in a cup and add 1/4 cup of the 2% milk, stirring until the cornstarch is dissolved.

After the onions are soft, add the curry powder, honey, salt, lite coconut milk, and remaining 2% milk to the skillet.

Stir well until the ingredients are well blended and then add the milk/cornstarch mixture.

Reduce the heat to medium-low and cook for about three minutes.

Add shrimp and simmer until they are opaque in center (about 5 minutes).

Serve the curry over rice and top with 1 tablespoon cilantro leaves per serving.

The refrigerator light goes on...
When I talk about Mediterranean diet I think about specific ingredients that go into a recipe – quality oils and fats, vegetables and seafood, for example. As such, those principles easily translate to so many different types of cuisine, and this Indian Shrimp Curry is a great example of how well Mediterranean diet principles translate to other cuisines.

Take some time to select your curry powder and try a few different versions. Some can be quite spicy and it is a good idea to add your curry powder a teaspoon at a time so that your recipe is not overwhelmed by too much curry powder.

Nutrition Facts	
Serving size	4 oz. shrimp w/sauce
Servings	4
Calories 220	Calories from Fat 72
	% Daily Value
Total Fat 8 g	10 %
Saturated Fat 5 g	19 %
Trans Fat 0 g	
Monounsaturated Fat 3 g	
Cholesterol 185 mg	61 %
Sodium 460 mg	20 %
Total Carbohydrates 16 g	6 %
Dietary Fiber 2 g	9 %
Sugars 8 g	
Protein 26 g	
Vitamin A 0 %	Vitamin C 6 %
Calcium 8 %	Iron 9 %
Vitamin K 6 mcg	
Potassium 500 mg	

Mushroom Risotto

Servings: 3 | Serving size: about 2 cups

Cooking time: 45 minutes

This recipe is easily multiplied by 2. This keeps well for a few days in the refrigerator.

2 tsp.	extra virgin olive oil
4 cloves	garlic (minced)
1 medium	white onion (diced)
1/4 lb.	crimini mushrooms (sliced)
1 cup	arborio rice
1/4 cup	white wine
2 1/2 cups	water
1/8 tsp.	salt
	black pepper to taste
1 oz.	dried shiitake, porcini, or portobello mushrooms (powdered)
2 oz.	semi-soft goat cheese
1 oz.	Parmigiano-Reggiano (grated)
10	grape tomatoes
2 tsp.	capers
6 large	leaves fresh basil (chiffonade)

Heat the olive oil over medium-heat in a medium sized stock-pot. Add the minced garlic and cook slowly. Do not allow to brown.

When the garlic is soft and translucent, add the onions and cook until they are also translucent. Add the button mushrooms and cook over medium-high heat until they begin to turn brown. Continue to cook, stirring continuously until the mushrooms are a dark roasted brown.

Add the risotto and cook for about 2 minutes, stirring frequently.

Reduce the heat to medium and add the white wine .Stir well. Cook for one minute and add 2 cups of water, the salt and pepper.

Cook over medium-heat, stirring frequently so that the rice will not stick to the bottom. After about 15 minutes, check to see if the rice is done. Add more water, 1/4 cup at a time as needed.

Slice the wild mushrooms.

When the rice is soft but not mushy, add the basil, wild mushrooms and parmesan cheese. Stir and cook for another 2 - 3 minutes over very low heat.

Serve topped with the julienne tomatoes.

The refrigerator light goes on...
Cooking mushrooms is not a timid enterprise. Because they are mostly water, mushrooms must be cooked until they begin to caramelize to bring out their rich flavor.

Nutrition Facts	
Serving size	about 2 cups
Servings	3
Calories 510	Calories from Fat 135
	% Daily Value
Total Fat 15 g	20 %
Saturated Fat 8 g	38 %
Trans Fat 0 g	
Monounsaturated Fat 3.5 g	
Cholesterol 25 mg	8 %
Sodium 530 mg	23 %
Total Carbohydrates 62 g	23 %
Dietary Fiber 7 g	26 %
Sugars 6 g	
Protein 21 g	
Vitamin A 0 %	Vitamin C 11 %
Calcium 4 %	Iron 17 %
Vitamin K 10 mcg	
Potassium 800 mg	

Roasted Salmon and Corn Relish

Servings: 2 | Serving size: 4 oz. salmon with relish

Cooking time: 30 minutes

Leftovers are great. I like to make sandwiches from the salmon and relish, but both go well chilled on top of salads.

Relish

1	red bell pepper
1 tsp.	olive oil
2 cups (~2 ears)	fresh corn kernels (frozen is OK)
1 small	shallot (minced)
2 clove	garlic (minced)
1 tsp.	fresh thyme leaves
4 Tbsp.	dry white wine
2 tsp.	lime zest
1	lime (juiced)
2 tsp.	honey
2 Tbsp.	fresh cilantro (chopped)
1/4 tsp	salt

Sauce

1 tsp.	olive oil
1/2	lime (juiced)
1 tsp.	honey
1/2 tsp.	paprika or smoked paprika
1/8 tsp.	salt

Fish

2	4 oz. salmon filets

Preheat oven to broil. Place the pepper in the oven and char, turning about every 3 minutes until black on all sides. Remove and place in a paper bag.

After about ten to twenty minutes remove peppers from bag. Peel, seed and set aside 1/2 of the pepper in the refrigerator for later. Cut the remaining pepper into 1/2-inch pieces.

Slice the white part of the green onion separate from the green tops.

Heat the grapeseed oil in heavy large non-stick skillet over medium-high heat. Add the corn, the white part of the green onions, the shallot and the garlic. Sauté gently until the corn begins to brown.

Add the thyme and white wine. Cook over low heat until the wine evaporates.

Stir in bell peppers, lime juice, honey, salt, the green tops of the green onions and parsley. Remove from heat. The relish can be made up to 24 hours in advance and reheated gently while the salmon is roasting.

Stir together the 1 Tbsp. grapeseed oil, lime juice, honey, paprika and salt. The sauce can be made up to 24 hours in advance.

When ready to serve preheat oven to 400°F. Line a roasting pan or skillet with foil. Place salmon in middle and top with the sauce. Place in the hot oven and roast for about ten minutes. While the salmon is roasting, gently reheat the corn relish. After ten minutes of roasting, remove the salmon and top each filet with 1/4 of the relish and garnish with fresh cilantro.

The refrigerator light goes on...
The amount of calories seems like a lot for a single entrée, but this includes the corn relish, which is a starch, and there are plenty of vegetables. Pair this with a simple salad and you have the perfect meal for a dinner party.

Nutrition Facts		
Serving size	4 oz. salmon w/relish	
Servings		2
Calories 420	Calories from Fat 108	
		% Daily Value
Total Fat 12 g		15 %
Saturated Fat 2 g		10 %
Trans Fat 0 g		
Monounsaturated Fat 4.5 g		
Cholesterol 60 mg		21 %
Sodium 520 mg		23 %
Total Carbohydrates 50 g		18 %
Dietary Fiber 6 g		21 %
Sugars 24 g		
Protein 29 g		
Vitamin A 19 %	Vitamin C 146 %	
Calcium 4 %	Iron 18 %	
Vitamin K 20 mcg		
Potassium 1300 mg		
Magnesium 61 mg		

Corn Quesadillas

Servings: 2 | Serving size: 1 quesadilla

Cooking time: 30 minutes

This recipe can easily be multiplied. Leftovers are sort of like cold pizza (an acquired taste).

1/2 tsp.	olive oil
1/4	poblano chili (seeded and diced)
1 ear	corn (shave kernels from the cob)
1/2 medium	red bell pepper (seeded and julienned)
1/4 tsp.	ground cumin
1/8 tsp.	salt
1 Tbsp.	cilantro leaves (chopped) spray oil
4	corn tortillas
2 oz.	Monterey jack cheese (shredded)

Heat the grapeseed oil in a large non-stick skillet over medium heat and add the chili. Cook for about 3 - 5 minutes until soft.

Add the corn and increase the heat to medium-high. Cook the corn kernels, tossing frequently, until they begin to brown.

Add the green onions and cook for about 3 minutes.

Add the red pepper, cumin and salt and cook for 5 minutes until the red pepper begins to soften.

Turn off the heat and add the cilantro and toss until blended into the vegetable mixture.

Preheat oven to 350°F. Place a large non-stick cookie sheet inside while the oven is preheating. After it is hot, spray the cookie sheet lightly with oil and place 4 flour tortillas on top of the cookie sheet.

Top each tortilla with the 1/4 of the corn mixture and then 1 ounce of shredded Monterey jack cheese. Place a tortilla on top of the corn and cheese forming the quesadilla. Spray very lightly with oil. Return the cookie sheet to the oven and turn on the broiler.

Cook for about 3 – 5 minutes on each side. Turn at

least once.

The refrigerator light goes on...
This is one of those recipes that wouldn't be possible without a non-stick pan and spray oil. The quesadillas that you get at Mexican restaurants are greasy because they use so much oil on the griddle (and no one is really paying attention to your arteries).

Nutrition Facts	
Serving size	1 Quesadilla
Servings	2
Calories 300	Calories from Fat 108
	% Daily Value
Total Fat 12 g	16 %
Saturated Fat 6 g	30 %
Trans Fat 0 g	
Monounsaturated Fat 4 g	
Cholesterol 25 mg	8 %
Sodium 340 mg	15 %
Total Carbohydrates 40 g	15 %
Dietary Fiber 5 g	18 %
Sugars 6 g	
Protein 13 g	
Vitamin A 12 %	Vitamin C 48 %
Calcium 24 %	Iron 8 %
Vitamin K 5 mcg	
Potassium 400 mg	

Jerk Shrimp

Servings: 2 | Serving size = 4 ounces shrimp and
1/4 cup salsa

Cooking time: 30 minutes

This recipe can easily be multiplied by 2, 3 or 4.
Leftovers are great in sandwiches and salads. The
Jerk Rub needs to be made beforehand.

Serve with Mango or Melon Salsa (recipe included),
lime wedges, and Coconut Rice (recipe included).

8 oz.	large shrimp (peeled & deveined)
2 tsp.	Jerk Rub
	spray oil
1/2 cup	salsa

Prepare the barbecue (medium heat) if the jerk is
to be grilled. If using a grill pan instead of using
a grill, preheat oven to 400°F and place the grill
pan inside.

Place the shrimp, grapeseed oil, lime juice and
jerk seasoning blend in medium bowl. Let marinate
at least ten minutes.

Thread shrimp onto metal or soaked wooden skewers.

Grill on the barbecue or grill pan for about 2
minutes on the first side and then turn. Cook until opaque in the center. Brush frequently with
marinade. Total cooking time will be about 5 - 7
minutes.

The refrigerator light goes on...
Bang, bang you're done. Keep some jerk rub in your
spice cabinet and you can toss it on shrimp or chicken
breasts. A little sweet salsa is easy to make and in 20
minutes you are ready to put on some Jimmy Buffett
and chow down.

Nutrition Facts	
Serving size	4 oz. shrimp with 1/4 cup salsa
Servings	2
Calories 123	Calories from Fat 18
	% Daily Value
Total Fat 2 g	3 %
Saturated Fat <1 g	2 %
Trans Fat 0 g	
Monounsaturated Fat 0 g	
Cholesterol 170 mg	57 %
Sodium 216 mg	9 %
Total Carbohydrates 2 g	1 %
Dietary Fiber <1 g	1 %
Sugars 0 g	
Protein 23 g	
Vitamin A 5 %	Vitamin C 4 %
Calcium 6 %	Iron 17 %
Vitamin K mcg	
Potassium 221 mg	

Jerk Rub

Servings: 24 | Serving size:1 teaspoon

Makes 1/2 cup

Keeps very well for months sealed tightly.

1 small	dried chipotle
1 Tbsp.	black peppercorns
1 Tbsp.	onion powder
2 tsp.	allspice
2 tsp.	ground cinnamon
1/2 tsp.	ground cumin
1 Tbsp	coriander seeds
1 Tbsp.	garlic powder
1 Tbsp.	ground ginger
1 Tbsp.	dried thyme
1/2 tsp.	ground nutmeg
1 Tbsp.	light brown sugar
1/2 tsp.	whole cloves
1 tsp.	salt

Combine all ingredients in a blender and blend on high speed until all ingredients are powdered.

The refrigerator light goes on...
There are a lot of dry rubs on the market very similar to this jerk. There's essentially nothing in them but flavor, so you can use almost as much as your spicy palate will allow. Many do have more salt in them than this recipe, so check the Nutrition Facts carefully.

Nutrition Facts	
Serving size	1 teaspoon
Servings	24
Calories 10	Calories from Fat 0
	% Daily Value
Total Fat 0 g	0 %
Saturated Fat 0 g	0 %
Trans Fat 0 g	
Monounsaturated Fat 0 g	
Cholesterol 0 mg	0 %
Sodium 100 mg	4 %
Total Carbohydrates 2 g	0 %
Dietary Fiber 0 g	2 %
Sugars <1 g	
Protein 0 g	
Vitamin A 7 %	Vitamin C 0 %
Calcium 0 %	Iron 0 %
Vitamin K 3 mcg	
Potassium 23 mg	

Chicken with Tarragon Mustard Cream

Servings: 2 | Serving size: 4 ounces chicken breast

Cooking time: 30 minutes

This recipe can easily be multiplied by 2 or 3. Left-overs are fair at best.

1 tsp.	extra virgin olive oil
2 – 4 oz.	boneless, skinless chicken breasts
1/2 cup	chicken stock
2 oz.	goat cheese
2 tsp.	coarse ground mustard
1/4 cup	2% milk
1/8 tsp.	dried tarragon

Preheat oven to 300°F.

Heat oil in a large non-stick skillet over medium high heat. Add chicken breasts and allow to cook for about 2 - 3 minutes, without turning. Then turn and cook for 2 minutes. (The surface should be seared brown on both sides.)

Remove the chicken and place on a sheet of foil to catch any juices and put in the preheated oven.

Deglaze the pan with the chicken stock and allow the sauce to reduce by about half.

Remove from the heat and add the goat cheese. Whisk in the cheese with the pan off of the heat until the sauce is smooth.

With the pan still off of the heat, add the mustard, milk and tarragon. Stir until the sauce is smooth.

Reduce the heat to low-medium and place the pan back on the burner. As the sauce slowly reheats remove the chicken breasts from the oven and place in the sauce. Turn frequently as the sauce and chicken breasts heat through (they are ready when the internal temperature is 160°F).

The refrigerator light goes on...
Rich, creamy sauces can be healthy. Start with less fat, cooking the roux carefully, stir constantly when adding the liquid and thicken with a lower fat creamy cheese.

Nutrition Facts	
Serving size	4 oz. chicken
Servings	2
Calories 271	Calories from Fat 114
	% Daily Value
Total Fat 13 g	20 %
Saturated Fat 7 g	35 %
Trans Fat 0 g	
Monounsaturated Fat 4 g	
Cholesterol 91 mg	30 %
Sodium 418 mg	17 %
Total Carbohydrates 3 g	1 %
Dietary Fiber 0 g	1 %
Sugars 3 g	
Protein 34 g	
Vitamin A 9 %	Vitamin C 3 %
Calcium 15 %	Iron 8 %
Vitamin K 2 mcg	
Potassium 409 mg	
Magnesium 47 mg	

Halibut with Seven Spices

Servings: 2 | Serving size: 4 ounces fish

Cooking time: 30 minutes

This recipe can easily be multiplied by 2 or 3. Serve with Rice and Lentil Pilaf (recipe included; make first). The fish makes good leftovers for sandwiches or salads.

1 tsp.	extra virgin olive oil
1 Tbsp.	pine nuts
2 Tbsp.	capers
1 large	tomato (seeded and sliced into julienne strips)
1/8 tsp.	salt
2 Tbsp.	balsamic vinegar
to taste	fresh ground black pepper
1 tsp.	unsalted butter
2 - 4 oz.	halibut filets (without skin)
1/8 tsp.	seven spice seasoning
	spray olive oil

Preheat the oven to 400°F. Place a medium or large skillet in the oven.

Place the olive oil in a medium non-stick skillet over medium-low heat. Add the pine nuts, capers and tomato and cook for about 2 minutes stirring once. Add salt, balsamic vinegar, pepper and butter and reduce the heat to low. Stir occasionally.

Sprinkle the halibut filets with seven spice seasoning.

Spray the hot pan from the oven lightly with olive oil and place the halibut filets in the hot pan seasoned side down. Return the pan to the oven and cook for about 4 - 5 minutes. Turn the filets and cook for another 4 - 5 minutes depending on thickness.

Remove and serve on top of Rice and Lentil Pilaf. Top with the tomato caper mixture.

The refrigerator light goes on...
This recipe is a great example of one that is higher in fat but low in saturated fat. While I try to keep Dr. Gourmet recipes under 15 grams of fat per serving, keep in mind that it is your average intake that is important. One day you might eat more and other days less. It is the long term reduction of fat, calories and cholesterol that can help you live longer and live better.

Those recipes that are higher in fat are like this one and have high levels of the healthy fats like monounsaturated fats and Omega 3 fats.

Seven spice seasoning is the best. Every time I open the spice drawer that I keep my ziplock bag full of this pungent spice in, the aroma evokes the market place and a spice merchant doling out small bags of spices. The market is crowded and loud with the bartering sellers and buyers. (Mind you, I've never been to such a place but the fragrance for the spice is so heady I feel that I know it.)

Nutrition Facts		
Serving size		4 oz. fish
Servings		2
Calories 229	Calories from Fat 103	
		% Daily Value
Total Fat 12 g		18 %
Saturated Fat 2 g		11 %
Trans Fat 0 g		
Monounsaturated Fat 4 g		
Cholesterol 41 mg		14 %
Sodium 469 mg		20 %
Total Carbohydrates 5 g		2 %
Dietary Fiber 2 g		7 %
Sugars 5 g		
Protein 25 g		
Vitamin A 20 %	Vitamin C 20 %	
Calcium 7 %	Iron 10 %	
Vitamin K 15 mcg		
Potassium 777 mg		
Magnesium 124 mg		

Mojo Pork Tenderloin

Servings: 4 | Serving size: 4 ounces pork

Cooking time: 60 minutes

This recipe can easily be halved or multiplied by 2. Leftovers are great for sandwiches.

2	navel oranges (juiced)
1	lime (juiced)
1 Tbsp.	fresh oregano (chopped fine)
1 tsp.	fresh thyme leaves
1 clove	garlic (minced)
1/4 tsp.	salt
1 Tbsp.	extra virgin olive oil
16 oz. (1 large)	pork tenderloin (well trimmed)
2 tsp.	unsalted butter

Mix together the orange juice, lime juice, chopped oregano, thyme leaves, minced garlic, salt, and olive oil in a large glass bowl.

Place the pork tenderloins in a zipper bag and add half of the marinade. Seal the bag and marinate at least overnight.

Place the remaining marinade in the refrigerator.

When you are ready to cook the pork, place a large skillet in an oven and preheat to 375°F.

While the pan is preheating, remove the marinating pork tenderloin and the extra marinade. Set the extra marinade aside.

Place the pork tenderloins in the preheated pan and return the pan to the oven.

Cook for 4 minutes and turn the pork every 3 minutes after that, until all the sides are seared.

Strain the remaining marinade used for the pork and discard the strained herbs and garlic, reserving the liquid. (If you do not strain the marinade, the herbs will burn and the sauce will become bitter.)

After the second turn, baste with 1/2 cup of the strained marinade, coating the tenderloins well.

As the pork cooks and the marinade is reduced, continue to baste the tenderloin to create a caramelized glaze on the pork.

It should take 20 – 25 minutes to reach an internal temperature of 140°F. As the pork is finishing, add the remaining marinade to create a syrupy sauce.

Remove the pork from the oven and place on a cutting board to rest for 5 minutes before carving.

While the pork is resting, add the other half of the marinade to the skillet, place the skillet over medium high heat, and bring the marinade to a boil.

Reduce the heat to a simmer and reduce the sauce by half.

Add the butter and whisk until smooth.

Serve the sauce over the sliced pork.

The refrigerator light goes on...
This recipe has so many valuable techniques. The marinade tenderizes and adds flavor while keeping food juicy. Braising is key to moist juicy meats. While this recipe uses a tender cut to begin with, tougher cuts of meat turn out well when braised. Basting helps create a rich glaze and the marinade makes a rich tangy sauce by slow reduction. All perfect over mashed potatoes.

Nutrition Facts	
Serving size	4 oz. pork w/sauce
Servings	4
Calories 190	Calories from Fat 72
	% Daily Value
Total Fat 8 g	10 %
Saturated Fat 2.5 g	12 %
Trans Fat 0 g	
Monounsaturated Fat 4 g	
Cholesterol 80 mg	25 %
Sodium 210 mg	9 %
Total Carbohydrates 5 g	<1 %
Dietary Fiber 0 g	0 %
Sugars 3 g	
Protein 24 g	
Vitamin A 2 %	Vitamin C 23 %
Calcium 0 %	Iron 8 %
Vitamin K 4 mcg	
Potassium 500 mg	

Tomato Saffron Risotto with Salmon

Servings: 2 | Serving size: about 2 cups

Cooking time: 30 minutes

This recipe can easily be multiplied by 2 or 3. This keeps well for about 48 hours in the fridge. Reheat gently.

1 cup	water
1 ounce	sun-dried tomatoes
1 tsp.	olive oil
2 cloves	garlic (minced)
1 large	shallot (diced)
1 large	leek (sliced)
1/2 cup	arborio rice
4 cups	water
1/4 tsp.	salt
1/8 tsp.	fresh ground black pepper
10 threads	saffron
1 oz.	Parmigiano-Reggiano (grated)
8 oz.	salmon filet (skinless, cut into 1/2 inch thick strips)

Heat the water in a small sauce pan. When the water is boiling add the sun-dried tomatoes and reduce the heat to a simmer. Let the tomatoes simmer for about ten minutes until soft. About have the liquid will remain. Remove and let stand. When cool puree in a mini chopper or blender.

Heat the olive oil in a large sauce pan over medium heat. Add the garlic and the green tops of the sliced leek. Cook over medium-low heat until the leeks begin to wilt. Add the shallot and the remaining leek.

Stir occasionally and after about 5 minutes add the rice. Stir for about one minute. Strain the liquid from the tomatoes into the pan and stir.

While the rice is cooking over medium-low heat place the sun-dried tomatoes in a blender or a mini chopper. Add 1/4 cup water and puree until a smooth paste.

Add more water to the rice as it cooks and evaporates. Stir occasionally. Add the salt, pepper and saffron. Continue to cook, stirring continuously and adding water gradually. Add the grated Parmigiano-Reggiano and stir until melted.

Taste the rice frequently checking for doneness. For this saffron risotto there should be more liquid and when the rice is stirred there should be about an extra cup of liquid. Add the flaked salmon to the risotto and stir gently for about 3 minutes and serve.

The refrigerator light goes on...
You can eat leftover salmon as long as it is cooked carefully. By cooking the salmon gently at the end of the recipe it won't be overcooked when the leftovers are reheated. Cook the leftover risotto very gently by heating on medium heat in the microwave for 90 seconds. Stir gently and heat for another 90 to 120 seconds until hot.

Nutrition Facts	
Serving size	2 cups
Servings	2
Calories 560	Calories from Fat 207
	% Daily Value
Total Fat 23 g	30 %
Saturated Fat 6 g	30 %
Trans Fat 0 g	
Monounsaturated Fat 7 g	
Cholesterol 75 mg	25 %
Sodium 640 mg	28 %
Total Carbohydrates 56 g	20 %
Dietary Fiber 4 g	15 %
Sugars 9 g	
Protein 36 g	
Vitamin A 16 %	Vitamin C 20 %
Calcium 14 %	Iron 17 %
Vitamin K 30 mcg	
Potassium 1100 mg	

Oven Fried Chicken

Servings: 4 | Serving size: 1 chicken piece

Cooking time: 30 minutes

This recipe can easily be multiplied by 2, 3 or 4. Leftovers keep well for 2 days. Allow to cool before refrigerating.

1	large egg
1	large egg white
1 Tbsp.	Dijon mustard
1 box (5 oz.)	plain melba toast
1 tsp.	dried thyme
1 tsp.	dried rosemary
1/2 tsp.	dried oregano
1/4 tsp.	garlic powder
1/4 tsp.	salt
1/2 tsp.	ground black pepper
1/4 tsp.	cayenne pepper
4 - 4 oz.	boneless, skinless chicken breasts
	spray oil

Place the egg, egg white and Dijon mustard in a small bowl. Whisk until smooth.

In a food processor fitted with a steel blade, place the melba toast, thyme, rosemary, oregano, garlic powder, salt, black pepper and cayenne pepper. Process until small breadcrumbs. Leave some pieces about the size of currants.

Preheat oven to 400°F.

Dredge a chicken breast in the egg mixture, coating thoroughly. Dredge in the breadcrumbs, patting and turning frequently until well coated.

Place the chicken on a cookie sheet or baking rack and then place in oven. Bake for 3 minutes and then lightly spray the top of each chicken breast with the oil. Bake 5 minutes more and then turn. Spray lightly with the oil again and bake for about 6 more minutes.

This recipe works well with any piece of chicken (with or without the bone). Use skinless legs, thighs or breasts.

The refrigerator light goes on...
Melba toast is amazing as breading! Fried chicken doesn't have to be fried to taste like fried chicken.

Nutrition Facts	
Serving size	1 chicken breast
Servings	4
Calories 293	Calories from Fat 36
	% Daily Value
Total Fat 4 g	6 %
Saturated Fat 1 g	5 %
Trans Fat 0 g	
Monounsaturated Fat 1 g	
Cholesterol 119 mg	40 %
Sodium 588 mg	25 %
Total Carbohydrates 28 g	9 %
Dietary Fiber 3 g	11 %
Sugars 1 g	
Protein 33 g	
Vitamin A 3 %	Vitamin C 3 %
Calcium 7 %	Iron 16 %
Vitamin K 6 mcg	
Potassium 412 mg	
Magnesium 59 mg	

Chili Rellenos

Servings: 2 | Serving size: 2 peppers

Cooking time: 60 minutes (chilling time not included)

This recipe can easily be multiplied by 2. Does not keep well.

4 medium	poblano peppers
1 tsp.	olive oil
1 small	chipotle in adobo (finely minced)
3 oz.	reduced-fat Monterey jack cheese (shredded)
4 Tbsp.	fresh cilantro (coarsely chopped)
1	large egg
1	large egg white
2 tsp.	Dijon mustard (or chipotle paste)
4 oz.	panko breadcrumbs
1/4 tsp.	ground cumin
1/2 tsp.	smoked paprika
1/2 tsp.	dried oregano
to taste	ground black pepper

Preheat oven to 350°F.

Place the poblano peppers in the oven and roast them for about 20 minutes. Turn them about every 5 minutes: the skin of the chili should begin to turn black and soften.

Remove the peppers from the oven and place in a brown paper bag. After about 30 minutes, the peppers should be cool. Remove them from the paper bag and gently peel the thin skin from the pepper.

Using the point of a knife, cut around the stem end and gently remove the core and seeds from the inside, trying to keep the pepper whole. Set aside.

While the peppers are roasting, place the olive oil in a large skillet and heat over medium high heat. Add the onion and cook for 7 to 8 minutes. Add the minced chipotle and cook for another two minutes.

Remove from the heat and chill the onion and chipotle mixture in the refrigerator for about an hour.

After the mixture is cool, toss it together with the cilantro and shredded cheese. Form the resulting mixture into 4 small cylinders. Place the cylinders inside the peppers and reform the poblanos to resemble whole peppers.

Place the egg and mustard in a small bowl. Whisk until smooth.

In a bowl, place the breadcrumbs, ground cumin, paprika, oregano salt and black pepper. Mix together with a fork.

Preheat oven to 400°F.

Coat the peppers with the egg and mustard mixture and then coat with the seasoned breadcrumbs. After all of the peppers are coated, place the peppers on a cookie sheet then put them into the oven.

Bake for about 7 minutes.

Spray lightly with spray oil and turn over, then cook another 7-8 minutes.

Serve immediately.

Nutrition Facts	
Serving size	2 peppers
Servings	2
Calories 480	Calories from Fat 135
	% Daily Value
Total Fat 15 g	20 %
Saturated Fat 9 g	43 %
Trans Fat 0 g	
Monounsaturated Fat 1.5 g	
Cholesterol 30 mg	10 %
Sodium 570 mg	25 %
Total Carbohydrates 60 g	22 %
Dietary Fiber 7 g	25 %
Sugars 10 g	
Protein 25 g	
Vitamin A 8 %	Vitamin C 218 %
Calcium 4 %	Iron 8 %
Vitamin K 30 mcg	
Potassium 600 mg	

Creamy Mac and Cheese

Servings: 2 | Serving size: 2 ounces pasta

Cooking time: 30 minutes

This recipe can easily be multiplied by 2 or 3. Left-overs are good. Reheat gently after adding 1- Tbsp. of 2 % milk per serving.

4 quarts	water
4 oz.	whole wheat elbow pasta
1 large	egg
1/2 cup	2% milk (1% milk will work)
2 1/2 oz.	reduced-fat cheddar cheese (grated)
1/8 tsp.	salt
to taste	fresh ground black pepper

Place the water in a medium stock-pot over high heat and bring to a boil. Add the pasta and cook until done. Do not overcook - the pasta should be cooked al dente.

While the pasta is cooking, combine the eggs and milk in a medium sauce pan. Whisk until smooth. Add the reduced-fat cheddar cheese and salt.

When the pasta is done, drain well and add it to the pot with the cheese over medium heat. Stir well until the cheese is completely melted and creamy. Don't let the mixture boil, and when the sauce is very thick, remove from the heat.

Add fresh ground black pepper to taste, stir, and serve immediately.

The refrigerator light goes on...
The key to this is to not overheat the sauce. The egg needs to cook, but if you let the sauce boil, it will likely curdle. That won't really affect the flavor, but the texture will be a bit lumpy.

Nutrition Facts	
Serving size	2 oz. pasta
Servings	2
Calories 350	Calories from Fat 99
	% Daily Value
Total Fat 11 g	14 %
Saturated Fat 5 g	28 %
Trans Fat 0 g	
Monounsaturated Fat 3 g	
Cholesterol 115 mg	38 %
Sodium 460 mg	20 %
Total Carbohydrates 44 g	16 %
Dietary Fiber 5 g	19 %
Sugars 3 g	
Protein 22 g	
Vitamin A 10 %	Vitamin C 0 %
Calcium 27 %	Iron 14 %
Vitamin K 1 mcg	
Potassium 400 mg	

Thai Coconut Shrimp

Servings: 4 | Serving size: 4 ounces shrimp

Cooking time: 30 minutes (not including marinating time)

This recipe can easily be multiplied. Leftovers are great. Keeps well for 24 – 36 hours. Serve over Coconut Rice (recipe included) with 2 tablespoons of Thai Peanut sauce (recipe included).`

1/2 cup	light coconut milk
2 cloves	garlic (minced)
2 Tbsp.	fresh lime juice
1 Tbsp.	fresh ginger (peeled & minced)
1 Tbsp.	low-sodium soy sauce
1 tsp.	hoisin sauce
1 Tbsp.	maple syrup
1 cup	Thai basil (finely chopped)
16 oz.	shrimp (peeled and deveined)

Place the low-fat coconut milk, minced garlic, lime juice, minced ginger, low-sodium soy sauce, maple syrup and basil in a blender and puree until smooth.

Put the shrimp in a zipper bag and add the marinade.

Seal tightly and place in the refrigerator for at least 3 hours (overnight is best). Turn the bag from time to time to redistribute the marinade.

When ready to cook, preheat the oven to 400°F.

Place a large skillet in the oven and let heat for at least 10 minutes.

Add the marinated shrimp to the skillet.

As they sear on one side, top the other with about half of the marinade.

The shrimp will grill fast and should be turned after about three minutes.

Spread the remaining marinade over the top of the shrimp and grill for another 4 – 5 minutes.

Serve over Coconut Rice with 2 tablespoons of Thai Peanut Sauce.

The refrigerator light goes on...

Roasting the shrimp in the oven is a perfect way to cook the shrimp, but they are also great on the grill. It is best to put them on skewers first. Use two skewers and arrange the shrimp like the rungs of a ladder before putting them in the marinade. This makes them easy to handle on the grill.

These shrimp are great served with the peanut sauce but are terrific as leftovers. They make great sandwiches or you can cut them up and toss them into salads.

Nutrition Facts	
Serving size	4 oz. shrimp
Servings	4
Calories 130	Calories from Fat 14
	% Daily Value
Total Fat 1.5 g	0 %
Saturated Fat 1 g	4 %
Trans Fat 0 g	
Monounsaturated Fat 0 g	
Cholesterol 185 mg	61 %
Sodium 300 mg	13 %
Total Carbohydrates 6 g	2 %
Dietary Fiber 0 g	0 %
Sugars 4 g	
Protein 24 g	
Vitamin A 0 %	Vitamin C 4 %
Calcium 7 %	Iron 6 %
Vitamin K 20 mcg	
Potassium 400 mg	

Salmon with Parmesan Crust

Servings: 2 | Serving size: 4 ounces salmon

Cooking time: 30 minutes

This recipe can easily be multiplied. The bread crumb mixture will keep well overnight, tightly covered. Leftover salmon makes great sandwiches or topping for salads.

1/2 cup	whole wheat breadcrumbs
1 ounce	Parmigiano-Reggiano (grated)
1 clove	garlic (minced)
1 Tbsp.	fresh basil (chiffonade)
1 tsp.	extra virgin olive oil
1/2 Tbsp.	balsamic vinegar
2 - 4 oz.	skinless salmon filets

Add the fresh breadcrumbs to a food processor or blender and process until they are fine crumbs.

Add the parmesan, garlic, basil, olive oil and vinegar and process until the mixture is well combined. This will make a moist breadcrumb mixture.

Place a large skillet in the oven and preheat to 375°F.

When the oven is hot, spread the breadcrumb mixture over the top of the salmon filets.

Place the salmon in the skillet and return the pan to the oven.

Cook for 5 minutes.

Set the oven to broil.

Cook for 3 minutes.

Serve.

The refrigerator light goes on...
This is a quick and simple recipe and relies on ingredients that you probably already have in your house – breadcrumbs, garlic, olive oil, and vinegar. You don't have to use salmon for this recipe. Almost any fish with will be complemented by the breadcrumb recipe.

The best part is that it is a super easy way to get a point on your Mediterranean diet score with a combination of seafood and the whole grain bread crumbs.

Nutrition Facts		
Serving size		1 salmon filet
Servings		2
Calories 390	Calories from Fat 198	
		% Daily Value
Total Fat 22 g		28 %
Saturated Fat 6 g		30 %
Trans Fat 0 g		
Monounsaturated Fat 7 g		
Cholesterol 75 mg		25 %
Sodium 350 mg		15 %
Total Carbohydrates 17 g		6 %
Dietary Fiber 2 g		7 %
Sugars 1 g		
Protein 30 g		
Vitamin A 12 %		Vitamin C 6 %
Calcium 10 %		Iron 3 %
Vitamin K 5 mcg		
Potassium 400 mg		

Fettuccine Alfredo

Servings: 2 | Serving size: 2 ounces pasta with sauce

Cooking time: 30 minutes

This recipe can easily be multiplied. Leftovers are fair at best.

1 tsp.	extra virgin olive oil
2 cloves	roasted garlic
2 tsp.	all purpose white flour
3/4 cup	2% milk (chilled)
1 ounce	semi-soft goat cheese
1 ounce	Parmigiano-Reggiano (grated)
4 quarts	water
4 ounces	whole wheat fettuccine
1 Tbsp.	fresh Italian or curly parsley (minced)

Heat the olive oil in a ten-inch non-stick skillet over medium heat and add the roasted garlic. Cook very slowly and stir frequently. Do not allow the garlic to brown or it will become bitter.

Add the flour slowly and cook for about one minute. Stir continuously to blend the oil and flour. The mixture will be like coarse corn meal. Cook gently so the mixture doesn't brown.

Slowly add the cold milk whisking to keep the sauce from forming clumps. Blend in all of the milk until the sauce is smooth and begins to thicken.

Add the goat cheese and whisk as it melts. When the sauce is smooth add the Parmigiano-Reggiano and whisk as it melts until the sauce is creamy. Reduce the heat to very low.

In a large pot heat the water to a boil. Add the fettuccine and cook until just tender (about 12 - 15 minutes for dried pasta). Drain well and then add the pasta to the sauce, tossing to coat thoroughly. Sprinkle the minced parsley over the top and serve.

The refrigerator light goes on...

Keep in mind a serving of any pasta is two ounces. I prefer to use the best quality Parmesan cheese and grate it fresh. By using the best quality ingredients you don't need as much to get maximum flavor.

Nutrition Facts	
Serving size	2 oz. pasta
Servings	2
Calories 389	Calories from Fat 107
	% Daily Value
Total Fat 12 g	19 %
Saturated Fat 6 g	30 %
Trans Fat 0 g	
Monounsaturated Fat 5 g	
Cholesterol 23 mg	8 %
Sodium 337 mg	14 %
Total Carbohydrates 53 g	18 %
Dietary Fiber 5 g	20 %
Sugars 5 g	
Protein 20 g	
Vitamin A 7 %	Vitamin C 11 %
Calcium 36 %	Iron 16 %
Vitamin K 33 mcg	
Potassium 354 mg	
Magnesium 107 mg	

London Broil with Mushroom Sautéed in Cognac

Servings: 3 | Serving size = 4 oz. steak with about 1/2 cup mushrooms

Cooking time: 60 minutes

This recipe is easily multiplied, but steaks should be no more than about 1.5 lbs. Leftovers are great. Serve with Garlic Mashed Potatoes (recipe included).

1/2 tsp.	olive oil
3/4 Lbs.	small crimini mushrooms (halved)
1/2 cup	shallot (minced)
3 Tbsp.	Cognac (bourbon will do also)
6 Tbsp.	non-fat beef stock
1 Tbsp.	pure maple syrup
to taste	fresh ground black pepper
1/2 Tbsp.	unsalted butter
1 lb.	lean London broil (top round)
1/8 tsp.	salt
to taste	fresh ground black pepper

Preheat the oven to 400°F.

Place a 12 inch non-stick skillet in the oven for about ten minutes. Remove and add the grapeseed oil to the pan and swirl to coat the pan well. Add the mushrooms and shallots and toss until well blended. Return the pan to the oven. Check the mushrooms about every 5 minutes and toss well. Stir with a wooden spatula, if necessary.

After about 15 minutes, the mushrooms will be well browned. Add the cognac, beef stock, maple syrup, pepper and butter. Toss well and return to the oven. Cook for another ten minutes, to reduce the liquid by about half. Remove the pan and set aside.

Place a 12 inch non-stick grill pan or skillet in the oven at 400°F. Heat for about ten minutes. While it is heating, carefully sprinkle 1/2 of the 1/8 teaspoon of salt across the top of the steak. Grind black pepper across the top. When the grill pan is hot, place the steak in, seasoned side down. Return the grill pan to the oven.
Before turning the steak, sprinkle the remaining salt over the top.

Rare steak takes about 8 minutes on the first side and 6 minutes after the turn. Medium rare steak takes about 12 minutes of the first side and 8 minutes after the turn. Remove the steak from the oven and turn the oven off. Place the pan with the mushrooms back in the oven. Place the steak on a cutting board and allow it to rest for 3 – 5 minutes. When ready to carve, slice the beef very thin cutting across the grain.

Serve over Garlic Mashed Potatoes and top with 1/3 of the sautéed mushrooms.

The refrigerator light goes on...
Eating healthy does not mean that you have to eat chicken or fish all the time.

Nutrition Facts	
Serving size 4 oz. meat w/mushrooms	
Servings	3
Calories 327 Calories from Fat 114	
	% Daily Value
Total Fat 13 g	20 %
Saturated Fat 5 g	25 %
Trans Fat 0 g	
Monounsaturated Fat 5 g	
Cholesterol 72 mg	24 %
Sodium 217 mg	9 %
Total Carbohydrates 16 g	5 %
Dietary Fiber 1 g	3 %
Sugars 6 g	
Protein 29 g	
Vitamin A 10 %	Vitamin C 5 %
Calcium 4 %	Iron 18 %
Vitamin K 0 mcg	
Potassium 1075 mg	
Magnesium 47 mg	

Philly Cheese Steak

Servings: 1 | Serving size: 1 sandwich

Cooking time: <30 minutes

This recipe can easily be multiplied. This recipe re-
quires leftovers and should be eaten immediately.
This recipe is good using any leftover flank steak or
London broil recipe.

The refrigerator light goes on...
Recipes with flank steak or London Broil make
for a wonderful, lean and tasty dinner but
here's the bonus – leftovers.

	olive oil spray
1/2	medium onion (peeled and sliced)
1	mini baguette (2.5 oz. or less)
1 Tbsp.	non-fat mayonnaise
2 oz.	roasted flank steak or London broil (thinly sliced)
1/2 oz.	reduced-fat Swiss cheese (shredded)

Spray a non-stick pan with olive oil and place over
a medium-high heat.

After the pan is hot, add the onions and reduce the
heat to medium. Cook the onions slowly until they
are well browned. Set aside.

Preheat the oven to broil.

Slice the mini baguette lengthwise and place under
the broiler with the cut side of the bread facing up
until the inside is slightly brown.

Remove from the oven and spread the mayonnaise on the bread and top with the sliced flank
steak Top with the onions and then place the Swiss
cheese on top of the sandwich.

Return the sandwich to the oven with the cheese
side up and broil until the cheese is hot and melted.

Nutrition Facts	
Serving size	1 sandwich
Servings	1
Calories 395	Calories from Fat 123
	% Daily Value
Total Fat 14 g	21 %
Saturated Fat 4 g	19 %
Trans Fat 0 g	
Monounsaturated Fat 3 g	
Cholesterol 41 mg	14 %
Sodium 524 mg	22 %
Total Carbohydrates 43 g	14 %
Dietary Fiber 6 g	25 %
Sugars 9 g	
Protein 26 g	
Vitamin A 1 %	Vitamin C 8 %
Calcium 23 %	Iron 16 %
Vitamin K 26 mcg	
Potassium 495 mg	
Magnesium 84 mg	

Sea Bass with White Beans and Tomato Vinaigrette

Servings: 2 | Serving size: 4 ounces fish with beans

Cooking time: 45 minutes

This recipe can easily be multiplied but does not make very good leftovers.

1 1/2 cups	water
1 oz.	dried wild mushrooms (like porcini)
12	grape tomatoes (quartered)
1 Tbsp.	olive oil
1 tsp.	balsamic vinegar
1 tsp.	olive oil
1 slice	prosciutto ham (about 1 oz.) (diced)
1/2 cup	carrot (small dice)
1/2 cup	celery (small dice)
1/2 cup	white part of leek (small dice)
1 - 15 oz. can	white beans (drained and rinsed well)
1/4 tsp.	dried oregano
1/4 tsp.	salt
to taste	fresh ground black pepper
2 - 4 oz. filets	sea bass (or other fatty white fish like halibut)
	spray olive oil

Place the water in a sauce pan over high heat. When the water boils add the dried porcini mushrooms and reduce the heat until the water is simmering. After the stock has cooked for about 15 minutes remove the pan from the heat.

Place the cut tomatoes, 1 Tbsp. olive oil and vinegar in a small bowl and toss well. Place the vinaigrette in the refrigerator to chill.

Preheat the oven to 400°F. Place a large non-stick skillet inside while the oven is preheating.

Place the 1 tsp. olive oil in a medium skillet over medium heat. Add the prosciutto and cook, stirring frequently for about 1 minute. Add the carrot and celery and cook, stirring frequently, for about two minutes. Add the leek and cook for another minute, stirring frequently.

Add the white beans, salt, pepper and oregano.

Strain the mushroom broth into the skillet with the white beans and discard the porcini mushrooms.

Reduce the heat to simmer. Stir occasionally while the fish cooks.

Lightly spray the skillet in the oven with olive oil. Add the sea bass skin side down and return to the oven. Cook for about 6 minutes and turn the fish over.

While the fish is cooking divide the bean mixture between two plates. When the fish is done (about 5 minutes on the second side) place the filets on top of the beans. Top the fish with the chilled tomato vinaigrette and serve.

Nutrition Facts	
Serving size	4 oz. fish with beans
Servings	4
Calories 453	Calories from Fat 119
	% Daily Value
Total Fat 14 g	21 %
Saturated Fat 2 g	12 %
Trans Fat 0 g	
Monounsaturated Fat 8 g	
Cholesterol 54 mg	18 %
Sodium 604 mg	25 %
Total Carbohydrates 49 g	16 %
Dietary Fiber 14 g	54 %
Sugars 5 g	
Protein 37 g	
Vitamin A 130 %	Vitamin C 25 %
Calcium 15 %	Iron 25 %
Vitamin K 33 mcg	
Potassium 1407 mg	
Magnesium 154 mg	

Pepperoni Pizza

Servings: 1 | Serving size: 1 pizza

Cooking time: 30 minutes

This recipe can easily be multiplied. Leftovers are good cold for breakfast. This recipe requires Pizza Dough and Tomato Sauce be made first (recipes included).

1/4 cup	Tomato Sauce
1/4 cup	shredded part skim milk mozzarella
1/2 oz.	Hormel Turkey Pepperoni (about 8 slices)
1/4 recipe	whole wheat pizza dough

Pizza is best baked on a pizza stone but a cookie sheet will work as well. Place the baking stone or cookie sheet in an oven that has been preheated to 500°F. Allow the baking surface to heat for at least 15-20 minutes.

Using 1/4 of the pizza dough recipe (for each pizza), gently stretch into 8-inch rounds. Don't work too hard to get a perfectly round shape.

Once the dough is formed, place it on top of the hot pizza stone and top with 1/4 cup marinara sauce. Place the pepperoni discs on top of the sauce and top with the shredded mozzarella.

Bake for approximately ten to twelve minutes until the crust is golden brown.

The refrigerator light goes on...
This pizza is the real deal. If you don't want to make your own tomato sauce, using one of the bottled sauces works fine. The Newman's Own® Marinara sauce is a good choice and not too terribly high in sodium (it will add about 225 mg of sodium to this recipe). It has a good sweet flavor that's just right for pizza. You can also look for a low-sodium tomato sauce if you are on a salt restricted diet -- they are much easier to find these days.

Nutrition Facts	
Serving size 1 pizza (includes dough and toppings)	
Servings	1
Calories 422	Calories from Fat 82
	% Daily Value
Total Fat 9 g	14 %
Saturated Fat 4 g	22 %
Trans Fat 0 g	
Monounsaturated Fat 3 g	
Cholesterol 32 mg	11 %
Sodium 702 mg	29 %
Total Carbohydrates 66 g	22 %
Dietary Fiber 9 g	35 %
Sugars 8 g	
Protein 22 g	
Vitamin A 5 %	Vitamin C 13 %
Calcium 26 %	Iron 25 %
Vitamin K 4 mcg	
Potassium 528 mg	
Magnesium 109 mg	

Pizza with Dill Pesto and Potato

Servings: 1 | Serving size: 1 pizza

Cooking time: 30 minutes

This recipe can easily be multiplied but doesn't keep well. This recipe requires Whole Wheat Pizza Dough and Dill Pesto to be made first (recipes included).

1 quart	water
2	small red potatoes (about 4 oz)
2 Tbsp.	dill pesto
1/2 oz.	fresh mozzarella (cut into small dice)
1/4 recipe	whole wheat pizza dough
to taste	fresh ground pepper

Place the water in a stock pot over high heat. Bring to a boil and add the potatoes. Cook the potatoes until slightly tender. Remove and allow them to cool. Slice into rounds about 1/4 inch thick

Pizza is best baked on a pizza stone but a cookie sheet will work as well. Place the baking stone or cookie sheet in an oven that has been preheated to 500°F.

Using 1/4 of the pizza dough recipe (for each pizza), and gently stretch into 8 inch rounds. Don't work too hard to get a perfectly round shape.

Once the dough is formed, place the pizza dough on a floured peel and spread the pesto over the dough. Top with slices of potato and sprinkle with the mozzarella.

Place the pizza on the heated pizza stone and bake for about 12 – 15 minutes until the crust is golden brown.

The refrigerator light goes on...
This recipe uses fresh mozzarella and not the dry, shredded American type that pizza joints use. Fresh mozzarella is so rich and melts wonderfully. You'll love it with the Dill Pesto and potatoes.

Nutrition Facts	
Serving size 1 pizza (includes dough and toppings)	
Servings	2
Calories 502 Calories from Fat 116	
	% Daily Value
Total Fat 13 g	21 %
Saturated Fat 4 g	18 %
Trans Fat 0 g	
Monounsaturated Fat 6 g	
Cholesterol 14 mg	5 %
Sodium 453 mg	19 %
Total Carbohydrates 82 g	27 %
Dietary Fiber 11 g	43 %
Sugars 7 g	
Protein 18 g	
Vitamin A 11 %	Vitamin C 46 %
Calcium 18 %	Iron 27 %
Vitamin K 9 mcg	
Potassium 843 mg	
Magnesium 133 mg	

Baked Penne

Servings: 6 | Serving size: 1/6 pan

Cooking time: 60 minutes

I would not multiply this recipe. This recipe is a meal unto itself and requires no side dishes. Leftovers are great! They can be divided and placed in ziplock bags and frozen.

2 tsps.	olive oil
2 medium	yellow peppers (seeded and cut into 1 inch squares)
2 medium	red pepper (seeded and cut into 1 inch squares)
1 lb.	eggplant (cut into 1 inch cubes)
6 small	shallots (peeled and halved)
12 oz.	whole wheat penne
5 quarts	water
2 large	eggs
2 Tbsp.	fresh oregano (coarsely chopped)
1 ounce	Parmigiano-Reggiano (grated)
1/4 tsp.	salt
to taste	fresh ground black pepper
3 oz.	fontina cheese (shredded)

lace a 10 inch Pyrex dish in the oven and preheat to 375°F.

When the oven is hot add the olive oil to the dish.

Add the peppers, eggplant and shallots in a 10 inch Pyrex dish and toss gently for a few seconds.

Roast for 45 minutes. Stir the vegetables gently every 10 minutes.

After 30 minutes of roasting place the water in a large pot over high heat.

When the water starts to boil, add the penne.

Cook until slightly underdone (about 12 - 15 minutes).

While the pasta is cooking, place the eggs in a medium size mixing bowl and whisk until smooth.

Fold in the oregano, parmesan, salt, and pepper.

Drain the pasta and add it to the egg mixture.

Add the pasta mixture to the vegetables in the Pyrex dish and fold together gently until well blended.

Sprinkle the grated fontina over the top.

Bake at 375° for 15 - 20 minutes until the top is lightly browned.

The refrigerator light goes on...
This is a creamy version of a Baked Ziti recipe. It is a similar recipe and not many more calories. It is still pretty healthy, but if you are working on your weight you might eat a smaller portion.

Nutrition Facts	
Serving size	1/6 pan
Servings	6
Calories 430	Calories from Fat 135
	% Daily Value
Total Fat 15 g	20 %
Saturated Fat 7 g	37 %
Trans Fat 0 g	
Monounsaturated Fat 4.5 g	
Cholesterol 100 mg	33 %
Sodium 420 mg	18 %
Total Carbohydrates 56 g	20 %
Dietary Fiber 10 g	34 %
Sugars 8 g	
Protein 21 g	
Vitamin A 19 %	Vitamin C 141 %
Calcium 16 %	Iron 19 %
Vitamin K 9 mcg	
Potassium 700 mg	

Barbecue Chicken

Servings: 1 | Serving size: 1 piece chicken

Cooking time: 30 minutes (does not include chilling time)

This recipe can easily be multiplied by up to eight. Leftovers are great.

1 cup	low-sodium ketchup
1/4 cup	apricot jelly
1/4 cup	dark brown sugar
1/2 cup	cider vinegar
1 Tbsp.	Worcestershire sauce
2 tsp.	water
1/8 tsp.	hot sauce
1/8 tsp.	garlic powder
1/2 tsp.	dry mustard
1 tsp.	chili powder
1 tsp.	paprika
1 tsp.	ground black pepper
1 piece per serving	chicken (breast, thigh, drumstick) (skin removed)

Mix all ingredients, except the chicken, in a blender and chill overnight.

Heat grill to medium heat (approx. 350°F).

Dip chicken pieces in barbecue sauce and place on grill. Turn frequently, spreading the rest of the sauce on the chicken as it cooks.

The refrigerator light goes on...

Barbecue sauce is a funny thing. Religion for some and with good reason. The complexities of making a good sauce are debated endlessly. This recipe relies heavily on the brown sugar and jam to create a caramelized glaze on whatever you decide to use it on.

Sugar adds calories, plain and simple. If you are really watching calories there are a lot of sauces out there with fewer calories and are actually pretty low in sodium. I use them actually more often than I make my own. I look for ones that are low in both calories and sodium.

Nutrition Facts	
Serving size	1 piece chicken
Servings	8
Calories 217	Calories from Fat 15
	% Daily Value
Total Fat 2 g	3 %
Saturated Fat 0 g	2 %
Trans Fat 0 g	
Monounsaturated Fat 0 g	
Cholesterol 68 mg	23 %
Sodium 126 mg	5 %
Total Carbohydrates 21 g	7 %
Dietary Fiber 0 g	2 %
Sugars 18 g	
Protein 28 g	
Vitamin A 10 %	Vitamin C 13 %
Calcium 3 %	Iron 8 %
Vitamin K 2 mcg	
Potassium 482 mg	
Magnesium 43 mg	

Ginger Cilantro Flank Steak

Servings: 4 | Serving size: 4 ounces beef

Cooking time: 60 minutes

To multiply, make separate bags of marinade with steak. Leftovers are fantastic and make good sandwiches and salads.

1 lb.	flank steak
3 Tbsp.	fresh ginger (minced)
1 Tbsp.	dark sesame oil
1 Tbsp.	low-sodium soy sauce
1 Tbsp.	rice vinegar
1 Tbsp.	Z-sweet stevia or Splenda
1 tsp.	hot bean paste
1/2 cup	cilantro leaves

Combine the flank steak, minced ginger, sesame oil, soy sauce, rice vinegar, Splenda, red bean paste and cilantro leaves in a zipper bag. Close the bag and toss to coat the steak well.

Marinate at least four hours in the refrigerator (overnight is best).

When you are ready to cook the steak, preheat the oven to broil or start the barbecue grill on medium-high heat.

Lightly spray a broiler or non-stick grill pan or skillet with oil. Put the flank steak on the pan and place it under the broiler (or place the steak on the grill). Cook for about 8 - 9 minutes on each side for medium-rare.

Remove to a cutting board and allow the meat to rest for about 5 to 10 minutes prior to slicing. Carve the meat as thin as possible and serve.

The refrigerator light goes on...
Comparing this with the Garlic Lime Flank Steak shows how different a recipe can be, even though it uses the same cut of meat and the same technique—the only difference here is the marinade. This recipe is not especially spicy, but can be by simply increasing the amount of hot bean paste.

Nutrition Facts	
Serving size	4 oz. beef
Servings	4
Calories 206	Calories from Fat 95
	% Daily Value
Total Fat 11 g	16 %
Saturated Fat 3 g	17 %
Trans Fat 0 g	
Monounsaturated Fat 4 g	
Cholesterol 48 mg	16 %
Sodium 246 mg	10 %
Total Carbohydrates 1 g	0 %
Dietary Fiber 0 g	1 %
Sugars 0 g	
Protein 25 g	
Vitamin A 3 %	Vitamin C 3 %
Calcium 3 %	Iron 1 %
Vitamin K 8 mcg	
Potassium 427 mg	
Magnesium 30 mg	

Pizza with Thai Peanut Sauce and Scallops

Servings: 2 | Serving size: 1 pizza

Cooking time: 30 minutes

This recipe can easily be multiplied and leftovers are good cold for breakfast. Serve with red wine (but not at breakfast) and a good movie. Make the Whole Wheat Pizza Dough and Thai Peanut Sauce first (recipes included).

1 tsp.	extra virgin olive oil
1 large	leek (cleaned & sliced into thin rounds)
2 Tbsp.	Thai Peanut Sauce
1 tsp.	extra virgin olive oil
6 - about 6 oz.	sea scallops
2 Tbsp.	unsalted dry roasted peanuts (chopped fine)
1/2 cup	fresh cilantro leaves
1/2 cup	fresh mung bean sprouts
1/2 recipe (1/4 for each pizza)	whole wheat pizza dough

Pizza is best baked on a pizza stone but a cookie sheet will work as well. Place the baking stone or cookie sheet in an oven that has been preheated to 500°F. Allow the baking surface to heat for at least 15-20 minutes.

Place 1 tsp. olive oil in a non-stick skillet pan over medium high heat. Add the leek and reduce the heat to medium. Cook until the leeks begin to soften and brown stirring frequently. Add the peanut sauce and toss to coat thoroughly. Set aside.

While the leeks are cooking, heat the remaining 1 tsp. olive oil in a small non-stick skillet over high heat. When the pan is very hot, add the scallops to the pan. Sear on one side about 3 minutes and turn. Cook on the other side for about another three minutes. Remove to a paper towel to drain. When they are cool slice them in half so there are two discs for each scallop (a total of 6 discs per pizza)

Using 1/4 of the pizza dough recipe (for each pizza), gently stretch into 8-inch rounds. Don't work too hard to get a perfectly round shape.

Once the dough is formed, place it on top of the hot pizza stone and top each with one half of the leek mixture. Sprinkle 1-tablespoon of peanuts per pizza and top with 6 scallop discs (seared side up) and then 1/4 cup cilantro leaves per pizza.

Bake for about 10 - 12 minutes until the dough begins to brown. Top with 1/4 cup bean sprouts and cook for another 2 minutes.

The refrigerator light goes on...
I love this recipe and you don't have to make it with the Thai Peanut Sauce recipe. There are a number of good sauces on the market, and they are not too high in calories, fat or sodium. I will often substitute the Whole Foods brand when I make this pizza and it still comes in at about the same nutrition content.

Nutrition Facts	
Serving size 1 pizza (including dough)	
Servings	2
Calories 465 Calories from Fat 71	
	% Daily Value
Total Fat 9 g	13 %
Saturated Fat 2 g	7 %
Trans Fat 0 g	
Monounsaturated Fat 3 g	
Cholesterol 28 mg	9 %
Sodium 480 mg	20 %
Total Carbohydrates 74 g	25 %
Dietary Fiber 10 g	40 %
Sugars 9 g	
Protein 29 g	
Vitamin A 21 %	Vitamin C 18 %
Calcium 8 %	Iron 28 %
Vitamin K 39 mcg	
Potassium 768 mg	
Magnesium 173 mg	

Grilled Sage Lamb Kabob

Servings: 2 | Serving Size: 1 kabob

Cooking time: 30 minutes (marinating time not included)

This recipe can easily be multiplied by any amount. The marinade keeps well overnight.

2 Tbsp.	fresh sage
2 Tbsp.	fresh chives
1 Tbsp.	fresh lemon juice
1 Tbsp.	pure maple syrup
2 Tbsp.	dry sherry
1 Tbsp.	extra virgin olive oil
1 Tbsp.	dark brown sugar
1/4 tsp.	salt
8 oz.	lean lamb shoulder
2 cups	water
4 medium	red potatoes
1/2	medium white onion (peeled and halved)
1/2	red bell pepper
6	shiitake mushroom caps

Place the sage, chives, lemon juice, pure maple syrup, sherry, olive oil, brown sugar and salt in a blender and puree until smooth.

Cut the lamb into eight, one-ounce cubes. Combine the marinade and lamb in a zipper bag. Allow to marinate in the refrigerator at least four hours (overnight is best).

Place the water in a stock pot fitted with a steamer basket over high heat.

Cut the potatoes in half. Place the potatoes and the half onion in a steamer and steam for 15 minutes. Allow to cool.

Quarter the half onion and the pepper.

On a skewer, alternate: mushroom cap, lamb cube, quartered onion, quartered pepper and potato. Keep the marinade in reserve.

Cook kabobs over a hot grill. Turn about every three minutes and baste with the remaining marinade as the kabobs cook.

The refrigerator light goes on…
More proof that red meat is okay. Buy the best quality New Zealand lamb and trim it well. Pair it with good aromatic herbs, such as sage or rosemary, and you can't go wrong.

Nutrition Facts	
Serving size	1 lamb kabob
Servings	2
Calories 627	Calories from Fat 126
	% Daily Value
Total Fat 14 g	22 %
Saturated Fat 4 g	19 %
Trans Fat 0 g	
Monounsaturated Fat 8 g	
Cholesterol 69 mg	23 %
Sodium 420 mg	17 %
Total Carbohydrates 92 g	31 %
Dietary Fiber 9 g	36 %
Sugars 22 g	
Protein 33 g	
Vitamin A 80 %	Vitamin C 279 %
Calcium 5 %	Iron 25 %
Vitamin K 33 mcg	
Potassium 2741 mg	
Magnesium 137 mg	

Gnocchi

Servings: 2 | Serving size: 10 gnocchi

Cooking time: 30 minutes

This recipe can be multiplied by 2. Leftovers are fair at best. I have kept the gnocchi refrigerated overnight but they are not as good as when fresh. Serve with Dill Pesto or Tomato Sauce (recipes included). Nutrition information is for the gnocchi only.

10 oz.	Yukon Gold potatoes
6 Tbsp.	all purpose white flour
1 large	egg
1/4 tsp.	salt
1/8 tsp.	ground nutmeg
1/8 tsp.	ground black pepper
4 quarts	water

Peel the potatoes, rinse and cut into 1-inch cubes. Place a steamer basket in a large sauce pan. Add about 1 1/2 cups water and set the pan over high heat.

Steam the cubed potatoes until very tender (about 20 minutes). Remove the steamer basket and allow the potatoes to cool until they are no more than warm to the touch.

Force all of the steamed potatoes through a potato ricer into a large mixing bowl. (If you don't have a potato ricer, the potatoes must be chopped until there are no lumps. Do not over mash them or the gnocchi will be pasty.)

Add 3 tablespoons of the flour to the potatoes with the egg, salt, nutmeg and black pepper. Mix together using a fork. The mixture will take on a crumbly consistency. Add 2 tablespoons of the remaining flour and blend well.

Knead the dough gently until all the flour is blended in. Stop kneading when the flour is incorporated. After the dough is smooth, cut it into 2 equal pieces.

Place one tablespoon of flour on a cutting board and roll each piece of dough into a rope about as big around as your thumb. Cut the ropes in 1/2

inch pieces (about ten per roll) and then roll the dumpling over the tines of a fork to shape the ridges of the gnocchi.

Boil at least 4 quarts of water and add the gnocchi no more than 2 servings at a time (20 gnocchi).

As they float to the top of the water, they are done. Remove them and add to prepared sauce.

The refrigerator light goes on...
There are hundreds, maybe thousands, of gnocchi recipes. Most of the basic recipes, much like pasta, are mostly carbohydrates and are low in fat. There are recipes that contain all different ingredients – from mushrooms to cheese to pesto. Choose the ingredients that might add more calories carefully, but do choose them. Making gnocchi is great fun and, with a bit of practice, you can create light fluffy pillows to swim in your sauces.

Nutrition Facts	
Serving size	10 gnocchi
Servings	2
Calories 200	Calories from Fat 0
	% Daily Value
Total Fat 0 g	0 %
Saturated Fat 0 g	0 %
Trans Fat 0 g	
Monounsaturated Fat 0 g	
Cholesterol 0 mg	0 %
Sodium 320 mg	14 %
Total Carbohydrates 43 g	16 %
Dietary Fiber 3 g	9 %
Sugars 1 g	
Protein 7 g	
Vitamin A 0 %	Vitamin C 0 %
Calcium 0 %	Iron 6 %
Vitamin K 0 mcg	
Potassium 600 mg	

Tomato Sauce

Servings: 10 | Serving size: 1/2 cup

Cooking time: 120 minutes | Makes 5 cups

Keeps well in the fridge for about 4 – 5 days.

1 tsp.	olive oil
2 large	onions (diced)
6 cloves	garlic (minced)
2 – 15 oz. cans	no salt added diced tomatoes
2 tsp.	dried oregano
2 tsp.	dried basil
1/2 tsp.	dried marjoram
1/2 tsp.	dried thyme
3 cups	water
1/2 tsp	salt
2 Tbsp.	no salt added tomato paste

Place a large sauce pan over medium-high heat.

Add the olive oil and swirl to coat the bottom of the pan.

Add the onions and cook until they are translucent.

Stir frequently and do not allow them to brown.

Reduce the heat to medium and add the garlic.

Cook for about 2 minutes.

Add the tomatoes, oregano, basil, marjoram, thyme and water and reduce the heat to medium low.

Simmer for 40 minutes. Stir occasionally.

Remove from heat, add the salt and puree until smooth with an immersion or conventional blender.

Reheat gently before serving.

The refrigerator light goes on...
Making your own tomato sauce is super easy – the hardest part is dicing the onions and mincing the garlic which takes about 5 minutes. The rest of the cooking is simply stirring the pan a few times and then another couple of minutes to puree the sauce.

The flavor is fantastic. The slow simmering of the sauce brings out all the umami richness of the tomatoes. If I have it on hand, I like to use 1 cup of no salt added vegetable stock and 2 cups of water in this sauce. It brings a tremendous added richness to the tomato sauce.

This is a perfect way to ramp up your Mediterranean diet score with fruit (tomatoes) and vegetables (onions) along with great quality fats (olive oil). Serve this over a whole wheat pasta and you are good to go with a simple easy meal.

Nutrition Facts	
Serving size	1/2 cup
Servings	10
Calories 43	Calories from Fat 14
	% Daily Value
Total Fat 2 g	2 %
Saturated Fat 0 g	1 %
Trans Fat 0 g	
Monounsaturated Fat 0 g	
Cholesterol 0 mg	0 %
Sodium 21 mg	1 %
Total Carbohydrates 7 g	2 %
Dietary Fiber 2 g	7 %
Sugars 4 g	
Protein 1 g	
Vitamin A 4 %	Vitamin C 26 %
Calcium 5 %	Iron 9 %
Vitamin K 5 mcg	
Potassium 311 mg	
Magnesium 18 mg	

Mustard Seared Whitefish

Servings: 2 | Serving size: 4 ounces fish

Cooking time: 30 minutes

This recipe can easily be multiplied but does not make very good leftovers.

1 large	egg
3 tsp.	olive oil
2 tsp.	Dijon mustard
1/8 tsp.	salt
1/8 tsp.	paprika
1 Tbsp.	dried sage (crumbled)
to taste	fresh ground black pepper
2 - 4 oz.	whitefish filets (trout, cod, drum, tilapia)

Whisk together the egg, 1 teaspoon of the olive oil, Dijon mustard, salt, paprika, sage and black pepper until smooth. Put the mixture in the refrigerator.

Place a large skillet in the oven and preheat to 400° F.

While the oven is preheating rinse the fish filets and pat dry with a paper towel.

When the oven is hot add the remaining 2 teaspoons of olive oil to the pan. Dredge both sides of the fish in the mustard coating and place them in the hot pan.

Return the pan to the oven and cook for about 4 minutes on the first side. Turn the fish over. Change the setting of the oven to broil and cook for about another 3 - 4 minutes. Serve.

The refrigerator light goes on...
The one key to this recipe is that the pan be very hot because the egg wash sears onto the fish when it hits the pan. Timing is everything in making the perfect fish recipe. Have the fish ready and already coated on one side. Remove the pan from the oven, add the oil, and swirl it around the pan. Coat the other side of the filets and add them to the pan quickly.

Nutrition Facts	
Serving size	4 oz. fish
Servings	2
Calories 265	Calories from Fat 151
	% Daily Value
Total Fat 1 g	26 %
Saturated Fat 3 g	15 %
Trans Fat 0 g	
Monounsaturated Fat 10 g	
Cholesterol 171 mg	57 %
Sodium 301 mg	13 %
Total Carbohydrates 1 g	0 %
Dietary Fiber 0 g	1 %
Sugars 0 g	
Protein 27 g	
Vitamin A 5 %	Vitamin C 1 %
Calcium 6 %	Iron 13 %
Vitamin K 4 mcg	
Potassium 448 mg	
Magnesium 30 mg	

Pan-Seared Pork Chops with Savory Peach Marmalade

Servings: 4 | Serving size: 4 ounces pork with sauce.

Cooking time: 45 minutes

This recipe can easily be multiplied and makes good leftovers. Serve with Mashed Yams (recipe included).

2 Tbsp	olive oil
1	clove garlic (peeled and sliced)
2 tsp	dry rubbed sage
1 small	Vidalia (or sweet) onion (diced)
1 pound	peaches (peeled & sliced thinly)
1/2 cup	low sodium chicken stock
1/4 cup	water
1	lime (juiced)
1/2 tsp	salt
1/4 tsp	ground cumin
to taste	fresh ground black pepper
2 tsp.	maple syrup
2 tsp.	unsalted butter
4 4-oz.	boneless center cut pork chops
1/4	red bell pepper (finely diced)

Place a medium stainless steel or non-reactive saucepan over medium heat. Add 1 Tbsp. olive oil, garlic, and sage, cook for one minute, stirring frequently.

Add diced onion and cook for three minutes. Add sliced peaches and 1/2 cup chicken stock. Reduce heat to low. Add water, lime juice, 1/4 tsp. salt, ground cumin, and black pepper, and stir well. Cook, simmering gently, for 20 minutes, until peaches are softened.

Gently mash peaches with a fork until they're the consistency of marmalade. Add 2 tsps butter and set aside. Place a large skillet in oven and preheat oven to 375F.

When hot, sprinkle the remaining 1/4 tsp salt over the pork chops. Add the remaining 1 tbsp olive oil to the hot pan. Place the pork chops in the pan,

seasoned side down.

Put back in the oven and cook for 7-9 minutes, then turn. Cook for an additional 5-6 minutes. Plate each pork chop and serve, topped with the peach marmalade and sprinkled with 1/4 diced red pepper.

The refrigerator light goes on...
I love the flavor of peaches with pork. They seem so right together. The addition of the sage and onions makes this simple topping for pork just a bit savory. This is a good example of using fats that are good for you like the olive oil with just a little butter to enhance the flavor and texture of the cooked peaches. It doesn't take much -- just a bit to finish off the sauce.

Nutrition Facts		
Serving size	4 oz. pork with sauce	
Servings		4
Calories 309	Calories from Fat 146	
		% Daily Value
Total Fat 16 g		25 %
Saturated Fat 5 g		24 %
Trans Fat 0 g		
Monounsaturated Fat 9 g		
Cholesterol 67 mg		22 %
Sodium 354 mg		15 %
Total Carbohydrates 14 g		5 %
Dietary Fiber 2 g		7 %
Sugars 9 g		
Protein 27 g		
Vitamin A 11 %	Vitamin C 40 %	
Calcium 3 %	Iron 7 %	
Vitamin K 9 mcg		
Potassium 721 mg		
Magnesium 38 mg		

Turkey Burgers

Servings: 2 | Serving size: 1 1/4-lb. burger

Cooking time: 30 minutes

This recipe can easily be multiplied and cooked hamburgers are good leftovers.

8 ounces	95% lean ground turkey
to taste	fresh ground black pepper
2 tsp.	olive oil
4 tsp.	Worcestershire sauce
1/4 tsp.	dried thyme leaves
2	whole wheat hamburger buns
to taste	lettuce (if used, iceberg recommended)
to taste	tomato
to taste	onions

Place a large skillet in the oven. Preheat to 375°F.

Combine the turkey, pepper, olive oil, Worcestershire sauce ,and thyme leaves until well blended.

Divide into two balls and form each ball into a patty.

When the oven is hot, place the burgers in the skillet and return to the oven. Cook on the first side for about 8 to 10 minutes.

Turn the patties over and return to the oven, cooking for an additional 5 - 7 minutes.

Serve on a bun with lettuce, tomato, and onions.

The refrigerator light goes on...
Look for ground turkey that is 90 to 95 percent lean. Most of the ground turkey will be a mix between white and dark meat, but that is good because the dark meat brings more flavor to your burger. Because poultry is a bit drier to begin with, you need to add back some fat to make it taste great, but in this recipe that is in the form of great quality monounsaturated fat :the olive oil. Just a little adds a lot of moisture to your burger.

Plain turkey burgers may not have quite as much flavor as ones made using ground beef. However, using a little Worcestershire sauce brings an amazing umami flavor to your burger - you might even end up liking this better than a regular hamburger.

Nutrition Facts	
Serving size 1 burger, plain, with bun	
Servings	2
Calories 310 Calories from Fat 56	
	% Daily Value
Total Fat 8 g	11 %
Saturated Fat 1 g	6 %
Trans Fat 0 g	
Monounsaturated Fat 4 g	
Cholesterol 60 mg	21 %
Sodium 410 mg	18 %
Total Carbohydrates 26 g	10 %
Dietary Fiber 4 g	14 %
Sugars 4 g	
Protein 34 g	
Vitamin A 0 %	Vitamin C 0 %
Calcium <1 %	Iron 9 %
Vitamin K 5 mcg	
Potassium 400 mg	

Cocktail Sauce

Servings: 4 | Serving size: about 4 tablespoons.

Cooking time: 30 minutes (chilling time not included)

This recipe can easily be multiplied by 2 or 3. This keeps well for about a week in the fridge.

3/4 cup	no salt added ketchup
3 Tbsp.	prepared horseradish
2 Tbsp.	fresh lemon juice
1/4 tsp.	Tabasco sauce
1/ tsp.	salt
to taste	fresh ground black pepper

Mix all ingredients together until well blended.

Chill for at least an hour before serving.

The refrigerator light goes on...
This is a good example of using a low-sodium food and then adding a measured amount of salt to the recipe for flavor. This allows you to better control the total amount of salt in the dish.

Nutrition Facts	
Serving size	1/4 cup
Servings	4
Calories 55	Calories from Fat 0
	% Daily Value
Total Fat 0 g	0 %
Saturated Fat 0 g	0 %
Trans Fat 0 g	
Monounsaturated Fat 0 g	
Cholesterol 0 mg	0 %
Sodium 191 mg	8 %
Total Carbohydrates 13 g	5 %
Dietary Fiber 1 g	2 %
Sugars 11 g	
Protein 1 g	
Vitamin A 9 %	Vitamin C 22 %
Calcium 2 %	Iron 2 %
Vitamin K 1 mcg	
Potassium 209 mg	
Magnesium 12 mg	

Thai Peanut Sauce

Servings: 8 | Serving size = 2 Tbsp. peanut sauce

Cooking time: <30 minutes

This recipe can easily be multiplied by 2, 3 or 4. This sauce will keep for about 3 weeks sealed tightly in the refrigerator.

1/4 cup	peanut butter
1 Tbsp.	low sodium vegetable stock (add more as needed)
1/4 cup	light coconut milk
2 tsp.	low-sodium soy sauce
2 tsp.	rice vinegar
2 tsp.	Tabasco sauce

Combine the reduced-fat peanut butter, chicken stock, reduced-fat coconut milk, low-sodium soy sauce, rice vinegar and Tabasco in a small bowl. Whisk until smooth and set aside. (This can be made up to 48 hours in advance and refrigerated).

The refrigerator light goes on...
Peanut sauce is a staple of Thai cuisine and using the lower calorie and lower fat ingredients makes this possible. These are ingredients that I always have in my pantry and you should too.

Nutrition Facts	
Serving size	2 Tbsp. sauce
Servings	8
Calories 60	Calories from Fat 54
	% Daily Value
Total Fat 6 g	7 %
Saturated Fat 2 g	11 %
Trans Fat 0 g	
Monounsaturated Fat 2 g	
Cholesterol 0 mg	0 %
Sodium 60 mg	3 %
Total Carbohydrates 2 g	0 %
Dietary Fiber 0 g	0 %
Sugars <1 g	
Protein 2 g	
Vitamin A 0 %	Vitamin C 0 %
Calcium 0 %	Iron 2 %
Vitamin K 0 mcg	
Potassium 65 mg	

Yellow Squash and Onions

Servings: 2 | Serving size: about 1 1/2 cups

Cooking time: 15 minutes

This recipe can easily be multiplied and makes good leftovers.

1 tsp.	olive oil
1/2 small	white onion (diced)
16 ounces	yellow squash (cut into 1/3 inch rounds)
1/8 tsp.	salt
to taste	fresh ground black pepper

Place the olive oil in a large skillet over medium-high heat.

Add the onion and cook for about 3 minutes until it begins to soften.

Add the yellow squash and cook, tossing frequently, for about 7 - 10 minutes.

Cook the squash only until it just begins to soften and then add the salt and pepper.

Toss for one minute more and serve.

The refrigerator light goes on...
I have loved yellow squash since I was a kid. For some this is strange but we ate a lot of veggies when I was growing up and my mother cooked great squash. The southern tradition was to cook it much longer, but I like squash that's not as overcooked as most people remember it. This recipe is quick and easy, full of flavor, and by not overcooking the squash it has great texture.

This recipe is a quick and simple way to improve your Med Diet Score for vegetables. This recipe is great with almost any fresh herb you might choose to add – especially dill and oregano.

Nutrition Facts	
Serving size	about 1 1/2 cups
Servings	2
Calories 70	Calories from Fat 27
	% Daily Value
Total Fat 3 g	4 %
Saturated Fat 0.5 g	3 %
Trans Fat 0 g	
Monounsaturated Fat 1.5 g	
Cholesterol 0 mg	0 %
Sodium 150 mg	7 %
Total Carbohydrates 10 g	4 %
Dietary Fiber 3 g	19 %
Sugars 7 g	
Protein 2 g	
Vitamin A 2 %	Vitamin C 50 %
Calcium 4 %	Iron 6 %
Vitamin K 8 mcg	
Potassium 500 mg	

Candied Carrots

Servings: 2 | Serving size: about one cup carrots

Cooking time: 30 minutes

This recipe can easily be multiplied and makes good leftovers.

2 cups	water
8 oz.	carrots (peeled and sliced)
1 Tbsp.	unsalted butter
1 Tbsp.	maple syrup
1/4 tsp.	salt

Place the water in a pot fitted with a steamer basket over high heat.

Steam for about 10 -15 minutes until the carrots are slightly tender.

Combine the cooked carrots with the butter, maple syrup, and salt and serve.

The refrigerator light goes on...
Most candied carrots recipes are way too sweet and the amount of brown sugar or molasses or maple syrup masks the flavor of the carrots. The combination of the unsalted butter and a small amount of maple syrup with the salt balances nicely with the natural sweetness of the carrots.

Nutrition Facts	
Serving size	about 1 cup
Servings	2
Calories 89	Calories from Fat 20
	% Daily Value
Total Fat 2 g	3 %
Saturated Fat 1 g	5 %
Trans Fat 0 g	
Monounsaturated Fat 1 g	
Cholesterol 5 mg	2 %
Sodium 224 mg	10 %
Total Carbohydrates 18 g	6 %
Dietary Fiber 3 g	12 %
Sugars 11 g	
Protein 1 g	
Vitamin A 365 %	Vitamin C 12 %
Calcium 5 %	Iron 1 %
Vitamin K 15 mcg	
Potassium 384 mg	
Magnesium 15 mg	

Coconut Rice

Servings: 2 | Serving size: 1/2 cup cooked rice

Cooking time: 45 minutes

This recipe can easily be multiplied and leftover rice can be used in stir-fries.

1/2 cup	reduced-fat (lite) unsweetened coconut milk
2 cups	water
1/2 cup	brown rice
1 medium	shallot (minced)
2 Tbsp.	cilantro (finely chopped)

Shake the can of coconut milk very well before opening. (Tip: a can of coconut milk will contain about 1 1/2 cups of coconut milk. Separate the remaining two 1/2 cups of coconut milk into two small ziplock bags and freeze for a later use.)

In a medium sauce pan, heat the coconut milk, water, and salt. When the liquid boils, stir in the rice.

Reduce heat to medium-low and simmer, covered, for about 35-45 minutes.

Do not boil away all of the liquid and do not stir the rice.

When a very small amount of liquid remains, remove the pan from the burner and let it stand, covered, for 5 minutes.

Just before serving, stir in the minced shallot and cilantro.

The refrigerator light goes on...
Never stir rice. It doesn't matter how you cook it, stirring it breaks down the starches on the outer layer and turns the rice to a gooey paste. Simply place the rice in the boiling liquid, stir once and cover. Leave it alone until the water is evaporated.

Nutrition Facts	
Serving size	1/2 cup rice
Servings	2
Calories 210	Calories from Fat 41
	% Daily Value
Total Fat 4.5 g	6 %
Saturated Fat 3 g	15 %
Trans Fat 0 g	
Monounsaturated Fat 0.5 g	
Cholesterol 0 mg	0 %
Sodium 150 mg	7 %
Total Carbohydrates 38 g	14 %
Dietary Fiber 2 g	7 %
Sugars 1 g	
Protein 4 g	
Vitamin A 0 %	Vitamin C 0 %
Calcium 0 %	Iron 7 %
Vitamin K 4 mcg	
Potassium 200 mg	

Jasmine Rice

Servings: 2 | Serving size: 1/2 cup cooked rice

Cooking time: 30 minutes

This recipe can easily be multiplied.

1 cup	water
1/4 tsp.	salt
1/2 cup	jasmine rice

In a medium sauce pan, heat the water and salt. When the water boils, stir in the jasmine rice.

Reduce heat to medium-low and simmer, partially covered, for about 15 minutes.

Do not boil away all of the liquid and do not stir the rice.

When a very small amount of liquid remains, remove the pan from the burner and let it stand, covered, for 5 minutes before serving.

The refrigerator light goes on...
Simple, simple, simple... When you add rice and salt to water and simmer and you don't stir the result is perfect.

Nutrition Facts	
Serving size about 1/2 cup cooked rice	
Servings	2
Calories 169	Calories from Fat 0
	% Daily Value
Total Fat 0 g	0 %
Saturated Fat 0 g	0 %
Trans Fat 0 g	
Monounsaturated Fat 0 g	
Cholesterol 0 mg	0 %
Sodium 293 mg	12 %
Total Carbohydrates 37 g	12 %
Dietary Fiber <1 g	2 %
Sugars 0 g	
Protein 3 g	
Vitamin A 0 %	Vitamin C 0 %
Calcium 1 %	Iron 11 %
Vitamin K 0 mcg	
Potassium 53 mg	
Magnesium 13 mg	

Herbed Zucchini

Servings: 4 | Serving size: about 2/3 cup

Cooking time: 30 minutes

This recipe can easily be multiplied by 2 using a large skillet. Leftovers are fair.

1 Tbsp.	olive oil
1 lb.	zucchini (cut into 1/4 inch dice)
2 Tbsp.	fresh herbs of your choice (minced)
1/4 tsp.	salt
to taste	fresh ground black pepper

Place the olive oil in a large non-stick skillet over medium-high heat. When the oil is hot add the zucchini. Let the zucchini cook without stirring for about 3 minutes. If it appears to be cooking too fast, reduce the heat to medium.

Toss the zucchini well and cook for about 7 - 10 more minutes. As the cubes begin to brown add the herbs, salt and pepper and continue to toss.

Do not over cook the zucchini. As soon as the outside is lightly browned and it is slightly soft, serve.

The refrigerator light goes on...
The choice of herbs here is not important. Use what you have in the garden or the fridge. Equal amounts of basil, chive, sage, rosemary and oregano will do but you could just as easily choose thyme, sage, marjoram and tarragon. This recipe will work with dried herbs, but it just isn't quite as good somehow.

Nutrition Facts	
Serving size	about 2/3 cup
Servings	4
Calories 51	Calories from Fat 32
	% Daily Value
Total Fat 4 g	6 %
Saturated Fat 1 g	3 %
Trans Fat 0 g	
Monounsaturated Fat 3 g	
Cholesterol 0 mg	0 %
Sodium 88 mg	4 %
Total Carbohydrates 5 g	2 %
Dietary Fiber 2 g	7 %
Sugars 2 g	
Protein 2 g	
Vitamin A 6 %	Vitamin C 33 %
Calcium 4 %	Iron 8 %
Vitamin K 26 mcg	
Potassium 321 mg	
Magnesium 23 mg	

Roasted Carrots with Fennel

Servings: 2 | Serving size: 4 ounces carrots

Cooking time: 30 minutes

This recipe can easily be multiplied and keeps well for about 24 to 48 hours in the refrigerator. Can be served hot or cold.

1 tsp.	fennel seed
1/2 tsp.	dried oregano
1/2 tsp.	dried basil
1/2 tsp.	dried marjoram
1/8 tsp.	black pepper
2 tsp.	olive oil
1 tsp.	honey
8 oz.	carrots (peeled and cut into 1/4-inch-thick sticks)
1/8 tsp.	salt
1 tsp.	honey

Place a small roasting pan in the oven and preheat to 325°F.

While the pan is preheating grind the fennel in a mortar and pestle or blend in a blender or mini-chopper until a powder.

Add the oregano, basil, marjoram and pepper to the ground fennel.

When the pan is hot add the olive oil and fennel mixture to the pan.

Swirl to coat the pan and then add the carrots, salt and honey.

Swirl the pan until the carrots are well coated.

Roast for 20 to 25 minutes.

Serve.

The refrigerator light goes on...
Fennel is a perfect flavor to combine with carrots. The subtle and slightly bitter flavor of the fennel is balanced beautifully by the sweetness of the carrots. Try this with a simple piece of grilled fish.

Nutrition Facts		
Serving size		4 oz. carrots
Servings		2
Calories 100	Calories from Fat 45	
		% Daily Value
Total Fat 5 g		6 %
Saturated Fat 0.5 g		3 %
Trans Fat 0 g		
Monounsaturated Fat 0 g		
Cholesterol 0 mg		0 %
Sodium 230 mg		10 %
Total Carbohydrates 15 g		5 %
Dietary Fiber 4 g		14 %
Sugars 8 g		
Protein 1 g		
Vitamin A 105 %	Vitamin C 8 %	
Calcium 5 %	Iron 5 %	
Vitamin K 20 mcg		
Potassium 400 mg		

Roasted Garlic Mashed Potatoes

Servings: 4 | Serving size: about one cup.

This recipe can easily halved or be multiplied by 2 or 3. These do not keep very well. This recipe requires Roasted Garlic (recipe included) to be made first.

3 quarts	water
1 lb.	yukon gold potatoes
2 tsp.	unsalted butter
1/3 cup	non-fat buttermilk
1/3 cup	2 % milk
1/2 tsp.	salt
4 cloves	roasted garlic

Place the water in a large stockpot over high heat.

Quarter the potatoes and add them to the stockpot. Cover with water by about an inch. Bring to boil and then reduce heat until the water is simmering.

Cook the potatoes about 15 – 20 minutes, until slightly soft in the middle. They should give when squeezed.

Remove from heat and drain water.

Add butter, buttermilk, milk, salt and roasted garlic.

Mash potatoes until creamy and the roasted garlic is well blended.

I like to leave some chunks of potatoes. If you like them smooth, be careful because over mashing will result in pasty potatoes.

Add ground black pepper to taste.

The refrigerator light goes on...
The key to good mashed potatoes is in the buttermilk / milk combination. The buttermilk adds richness and tartness, with little fat, and the milk adds creaminess. The butter is used here only as a flavor enhancer.

Nutrition Facts	
Serving size	1 cup
Servings	4
Calories 120	Calories from Fat 23
	% Daily Value
Total Fat 2.5 g	3 %
Saturated Fat 1.5 g	8 %
Trans Fat 0 g	
Monounsaturated Fat 0.5 g	
Cholesterol 10 mg	3 %
Sodium 370 mg	16 %
Total Carbohydrates 21 g	8 %
Dietary Fiber 2 g	7 %
Sugars 4 g	
Protein 4 g	
Vitamin A 2 %	Vitamin C 12 %
Calcium 5 %	Iron 5 %
Vitamin K 4 mcg	
Potassium 600 mg	

Roasted Parsnips and Carrots

Servings: 4 | Serving size: 4 oz. veggies

Cooking time: 30 minutes

This recipe can easily be multiplied by 2. These keep well for about 48 hours in the fridge and is good served cold at picnics.

8 oz.	carrots (peeled and sliced into rounds)
8 oz.	parsnips (peeled and sliced into rounds)
1 Tbsp.	olive oil
1 tsp.	dried rosemary
1 tsp.	salt
to taste	fresh ground black pepper

Place a large baking sheet in the oven and preheat the oven to 400°F.

Fold the carrots, parsnips, rosemary, salt, and pepper together and place on the baking sheet and return to the oven.

Reduce the oven heat to 375°F.

Roast the carrots and parsnips for about 20 to 25 minutes, stirring once or twice, until the carrots and parsnips are slightly soft and are lightly browned.

Serve hot or allow to cool and then refrigerate.

The refrigerator light goes on...
While this recipe is cooking your house will fill up with the lovely aroma of rosemary. Great hot or cold, take this dish to your next potluck: easy, colorful and delicious.

This recipe seems deceptively simple, and those are often the best dishes. The carrots and parsnips speak for themselves with great sweet flavors of the veggies that is made better with a bit of rosemary and the slight caramelization of roasting.

The instructions call for cutting the veggies into rounds, but if you have smaller carrots and parsnips or those that are fat at one end and tapered at the other, cut full rounds at the tapered end and half or quarter rounds depending on the size at the base. The goal is to have your cut carrots and parsnips all about the same size.

Nutrition Facts	
Serving size	4 oz. veggies
Servings	4
Calories 100	Calories from Fat 32
	% Daily Value
Total Fat 3.5 g	5 %
Saturated Fat 0.5 g	3 %
Trans Fat 0 g	
Monounsaturated Fat 2.5 g	
Cholesterol 0 mg	0 %
Sodium 120 mg	5 %
Total Carbohydrates 16 g	6 %
Dietary Fiber 4 g	16 %
Sugars 5 g	
Protein 1 g	
Vitamin A 53 %	Vitamin C 14 %
Calcium 3 %	Iron 3 %
Vitamin K 20 mcg	
Potassium 400 mg	

French Fries

Servings: 4 | Serving size: about 6 ounces fries

Cooking time: 45 minutes

This recipe can easily be multiplied by 2, but must be cooked in two batches. These do not keep very well at all.

24 oz.	russet potatoes (peeled and cut into 1/4 inch strips)
6 quarts	water
4 tsp.	baking powder
2 tsp.	olive oil
1/8 tsp.	salt

Place the water in a large sauce pan over high heat.

While the water is coming to a boil, peel and cut the potatoes into 1/4 inch by 1/4 inch strips.

When the water begins to boil reduce the heat to a simmer and add the baking powder while stirring gently. The water will foam slightly.

Add the potatoes and stir gently.

Let the potatoes cook for 10 minutes.

Remove and let the potatoes cool.

Place a large cookie sheet (preferably non-stick) in the oven.

Preheat the oven to 400°F.

When the oven is hot, add the olive oil to the cookie sheet and then the potatoes.

Toss to coat well and then roast for 30 minutes. Shake the pan every 10 minutes.

Serve immediately topped with the salt.

The refrigerator light goes on...
Oven fried foods are just like deep fried ones, if you handle them right. Most of the time, you have to eat the dish right away. These French Fries, for instance, will keep for all of about 20 minutes (about the same amount of time as ones that have been deep fried).

This technique of precooking the potatoes in the water with the baking powder works wonders. The baking powder contains some cornstarch along with both baking soda and either sodium acid pyrophosphate or sodium aluminum sulfate. These three work well to create a coating on the outside of the potato that helps them crisp better and is definitely worth taking the extra step.

The best part is that your own French Fries are lower in calories and contain much better quality of fats: these French Fries have 170 calories, 2.5 grams of fat, no saturated fat, 1.5 grams of monounsaturated fat, and 3 grams of fiber, while Fast Food Fries have 220 calories, 10 grams of fat, 2.5 grams of saturated fat, and 3 grams of fiber (the amount of monounsaturated fat is not reported).

Nutrition Facts		
Serving size		6 oz. fries
Servings		4
Calories 170	Calories from Fat 23	
		% Daily Value
Total Fat 2.5 g		3 %
Saturated Fat 0 g		0 %
Trans Fat 0 g		
Monounsaturated Fat 1.5 g		
Cholesterol 0 mg		0 %
Sodium 200 mg		9 %
Total Carbohydrates 34 g		12 %
Dietary Fiber 3 g		11 %
Sugars 2 g		
Protein 3 g		
Vitamin A 0 %	Vitamin C 14 %	
Calcium 6 %	Iron 4 %	
Vitamin K 5 mcg		
Potassium 600 mg		

Roasted Beets

Servings: 4 | Serving size: about 1 cup beets

Cooking time: 30 minutes

This recipe can easily be multiplied but a larger roasting pan must be used. Leftovers are great ingredients in tossed salads.

2	medium beets
1 tsp.	unsalted butter
1/4 tsp.	salt
1/8 tsp.	dried oregano
1/8 tsp.	chili powder

Preheat the oven to 400°F.

Wrap beets in a paper towel and cook on high in microwave for 5 minutes. Let cool for 5 minutes.

Peel and cut into 1 inch cubes.

Place in a roasting pan large enough so that the beets are not completely touching.

Put the pat of butter on the beets and sprinkle the salt, oregano and chili powder over the top.

Reduce the heat to 375°F and roast for 20 – 25 minutes. The beets are done when they are slightly crisp on the outside.

The refrigerator light goes on...
Roasting is an essential technique in cooking great healthy food. The most important thing is that the roasting pan be large enough so that the food doesn't touch. If you use too small a pan, the food will steam and not have that crispy outside the makes roasted food so great.

Nutrition Facts	
Serving size	1 cup
Servings	2
Calories 25	Calories from Fat 9
	% Daily Value
Total Fat 1 g	0 %
Saturated Fat 0.5 g	3 %
Trans Fat 0 g	
Monounsaturated Fat 0 g	
Cholesterol <5 mg	0 %
Sodium 180 mg	8 %
Total Carbohydrates 4 g	0 %
Dietary Fiber 1 g	4 %
Sugars 3 g	
Protein <1 g	
Vitamin A 0 %	Vitamin C 2 %
Calcium 0 %	Iron 2 %
Vitamin K 0 mcg	
Potassium 100 mg	

Roasted Acorn Squash

Servings: 2 | Serving size: 1/2 squash

Cooking time: 45 minutes

This recipe can be easily multiplied. The leftovers make a good ingredient in tossed salads.

1	acorn squash (about 1 pound)
1 tsp.	butter
2 tsp.	brown sugar

Preheat oven to 400°F.

Halve the squash lengthwise. Scoop out the seeds and discard them. Make shallow cuts in a grid pattern along the inside of the squash.

Place 1/2 tsp. butter and 1/2 tsp. brown sugar in the cavity of each squash.

Set the squash in the preheated oven and reduce the heat to 350°F. Roast for approximately 30 minutes. Using a spoon occasionally baste the top and inside of the squash with the sugar/butter mixture.

Remove and serve after allowing to cool for about 5 minutes.

The refrigerator light goes on...
Simple dishes are the best. Pair this roasted acorn squash with a roasted salmon dish and you have the nearly perfect meal.

Nutrition Facts		
Serving size		1/2 squash
Servings		2
Calories 120	Calories from Fat 18	
		% Daily Value
Total Fat 2 g		3 %
Saturated Fat 1 g		6 %
Trans Fat 0 g		
Monounsaturated Fat 0.5 g		
Cholesterol 5 mg		0 %
Sodium 10 mg		0 %
Total Carbohydrates 27 g		10 %
Dietary Fiber 3 g		12 %
Sugars 4 g		
Protein 2 g		
Vitamin A 6 %	Vitamin C 26 %	
Calcium 6 %	Iron 9 %	
Vitamin K 0 mcg		
Potassium 800 mg		

Brown Rice

Servings: 2 | Serving size: 1/2 cup cooked rice

Cooking time: 45 minutes

This recipe can easily be multiplied and keeps well.

2 1/4 cups	water
1/4 tsp.	salt
1/2 cup	long grain brown rice

In a medium sauce pan, heat the water and salt. When the water boils, stir in the brown rice.

Reduce heat to medium-low and simmer, partially covered, for 30 -- 35 minutes.

Do not boil away all of the liquid and do not stir the rice.

When a very small amount of liquid remains, re-move the pan from the burner and let it stand, covered, for 5 minutes before serving.

The refrigerator light goes on...
Simple, simple, simple... When you add rice and salt to water and simmer and you don't stir the result is perfect.

Nutrition Facts	
Serving size about 1/2 cup cooked rice	
Servings	2
Calories 170	Calories from Fat 14
	% Daily Value
Total Fat 1.5 g	0 %
Saturated Fat 0 g	0 %
Trans Fat 0 g	
Monounsaturated Fat 0 g	
Cholesterol 0 mg	0 %
Sodium 300 mg	13 %
Total Carbohydrates 35 g	13 %
Dietary Fiber 2 g	6 %
Sugars 0 g	
Protein 3 g	
Vitamin A 0 %	Vitamin C 0 %
Calcium 0 %	Iron 3 %
Vitamin K 0 mcg	
Potassium 100 mg	

Plain Mashed Potatoes

Servings: 4 | Serving size: about one cup

Cooking time: 30 minutes

This recipe can easily be multiplied. Leftovers are fair. Reheat gently.

3 quarts	water
1 lb.	yukon gold potatoes
2 tsp.	unsalted butter
1/4 cup	reduced-fat buttermilk
1/4 cup	2 % milk
1/4 tsp.	salt
to taste	fresh ground black pepper

Place the water in a large stock pot over high heat.

Quarter the potatoes and add to the stock pot. Cover with water by about an inch. Bring to boil and then reduce heat until the water is simmering.

Cook the potatoes about 15 – 20 minutes until slightly soft in the middle. They should give when squeezed.

Remove from heat and drain water. Add butter, buttermilk, milk and salt. Mash potatoes until creamy. I like to leave some chunks. If you like them smooth, be careful because over mashing will result in pasty potatoes. Add ground black pepper to taste.

The refrigerator light goes on...
These potatoes have more butter in them than some of the other "flavored" mashed potato recipes in this book. This is to help enhance the creaminess and the mouthfeel that other flavors, like roasted garlic, achieve with less fat.

Nutrition Facts	
Serving size	1 cup
Servings	4
Calories 110	Calories from Fat 23
	% Daily Value
Total Fat 2.5 g	3 %
Saturated Fat 1.5 g	8 %
Trans Fat 0 g	
Monounsaturated Fat 0.5 g	
Cholesterol 5 mg	2 %
Sodium 200 mg	9 %
Total Carbohydrates 19 g	7 %
Dietary Fiber 3 g	10 %
Sugars 3 g	
Protein 3 g	
Vitamin A 2 %	Vitamin C 12 %
Calcium 4 %	Iron 3 %
Vitamin K 2 mcg	
Potassium 500 mg	

Roasted Corn on the Cob

Servings: 2 | Serving size: 1 ear corn

Cooking time: 45 minutes

This recipe is easily multiplied. I love leftover corn. Leave it wrapped in the husks inside the foil.

2 ears	corn
1/8 tsp.	pepper
1/4 tsp.	salt
2 tsp.	unsalted butter

Preheat the oven to 400°F.

Peel the husk back from the corn, being careful not to detach them from the stem. Remove silks and rinse well, wetting down the husks.

Sprinkle the salt and pepper over the corn.

Fold the husks against the corn and wrap in foil.

Roast in the oven for about 30 minutes. Turn them 1/4 turn about every 7 - 8 minutes.

Remove from the oven and unwrap the foil. Cut the bottom of the cob so that the husks fall away easily.

Serve each with a pat of butter.

These can also be roasted on top of the grill. The heat should be medium to medium-high and you must turn them frequently, as noted above.

The refrigerator light goes on...
This recipe includes the pat of butter for your corn on the cob because it just wouldn't be corn without it. Take the pat and enjoy it. This recipe works well both on the grill and in the oven. The grill will give the corn a lovely charcoal flavor.

Nutrition Facts	
Serving size	1 ear
Servings	2
Calories 160	Calories from Fat 54
	% Daily Value
Total Fat 6 g	7 %
Saturated Fat 3 g	14 %
Trans Fat 0 g	
Monounsaturated Fat 1.5 g	
Cholesterol 10 mg	3 %
Sodium 320 mg	14 %
Total Carbohydrates 27 g	10 %
Dietary Fiber 3 g	10 %
Sugars 9 g	
Protein 5 g	
Vitamin A 5 %	Vitamin C 11 %
Calcium 0 %	Iron 4 %
Vitamin K 1 mcg	
Potassium 400 mg	

Parmesan Squash

Servings: 2 | Serving size: 1 8-oz. squash

Cooking time: 30 minutes

This recipe can easily be multiplied and leftovers are fair. Chilled, they make great additions to salads.

2 large (8 oz./ea.)	yellow squash
2 cups	water
to taste	fresh ground black pepper
2 Tbsp.	fresh herbs of your choice (minced)
1 oz.	Parmigiano-reggiano (grated)

Place the water in a medium pot fitted with a steamer basket over high heat.

Preheat the oven to 325°F.

Cut about 1/4 inch from the stem end of the squash and then slice lengthwise. Place the four halves in the steamer and steam until slightly tender.

Remove the steamed squash and place in a shallow baking dish. Place the dish in the oven and cook for about 10 minutes. Remove and sprinkle with pepper, fresh herbs and equal amounts of Parmigiano-reggiano.

Return the pan to the oven and cook until the parmesan is melted (about 5 minutes).

The refrigerator light goes on...
These are two delicious ingredients that make a wonderful dish. The yellow squash tastes like summer, and its own buttery flavor is enhanced by the parmesan. I especially like using just a little bit of rosemary for the herb, and that's what was used to calculate the Nutrition Facts.

Nutrition Facts	
Serving size	1 large squash
Servings	2
Calories 110	Calories from Fat 41
	% Daily Value
Total Fat 4.5 g	6 %
Saturated Fat 2.5 g	12 %
Trans Fat 0 g	
Monounsaturated Fat 1 g	
Cholesterol 10 mg	4 %
Sodium 260 mg	11 %
Total Carbohydrates 11 g	4 %
Dietary Fiber 3 g	9 %
Sugars 7 g	
Protein 6 g	
Vitamin A 6 %	Vitamin C 49 %
Calcium 13 %	Iron 7 %
Vitamin K 8 mcg	
Potassium 500 mg	

ab/

Melon Salsa

Servings: 8 | Serving Size = 1/4 cup (makes 2 cups)

Cooking time: 30 minutes (does not include chilling time)

This recipe can be halved or multiplied and keeps in the refrigerator for 48 hours.

6 oz.	cantaloupe (diced)
4 oz.	honeydew melon (diced)
1/4 cup	red onion (diced)
1/4 cup	fresh cilantro (chopped)
1 Tbsp.	fresh lime juice
1/8 tsp.	salt
1/8 tsp.	chili powder

Fold together the cantaloupe, honeydew, red onion, cilantro, lime juice, salt, and chili powder.

Chill at least 4 hours.

The refrigerator light goes on...
This recipe is a variation on a fruit salsa recipe we created with mango. Melon is likely easier to find, and this is a great way to try your own combination of fruits in salsa!

Nutrition Facts	
Serving size	1/4 cup
Servings	8
Calories 15	Calories from Fat 0
	% Daily Value
Total Fat 0 g	0 %
Saturated Fat 0 g	0 %
Trans Fat 0 g	
Monounsaturated Fat 0 g	
Cholesterol 0 mg	0 %
Sodium 45 mg	0 %
Total Carbohydrates 4 g	0 %
Dietary Fiber 0 g	2 %
Sugars 3 g	
Protein 0 g	
Vitamin A 4 %	Vitamin C 13 %
Calcium 0 %	Iron 1 %
Vitamin K 3 mcg	
Potassium 100 mg	

The Dr. Gourmet Diet for Coumadin Users
111/

Couscous

Servings: 4 | Serving size: about 1/2 cup cooked

Cooking time: 30 minutes

This recipe can easily be multiplied or divided by 2. Keeps well for about 48 hours.

2 cups	water
1/4 tsp.	salt
1 cup	couscous
1 tsp.	olive oil
1/2 cup	dried currants
1	green onion (minced)
1 Tbsp.	flat leaf parsley (chopped fine)
1 Tbsp.	fresh basil (chopped fine)

Place water and salt in a medium sized pan over high heat and bring to a boil. Remove from the heat and add couscous, stirring once. Cover and let stand for five minutes.

As the couscous is cooking, place the oil in a small non-stick sauté pan over medium heat. Add the currants and green onion. Cook, stirring occasionally.

After the couscous has stood for five minutes, remove the top and fluff with a fork. Add the currant and green onion mixture, parsley and basil and toss well.

The refrigerator light goes on...
Couscous is the perfect pantry item. It keeps almost forever. It is simple to make, taking all of 5 minutes to cook and you can put almost anything in it to make it exotic.

Nutrition Facts	
Serving size	1/2 cup cooked
Servings	4
Calories 230	Calories from Fat 14
	% Daily Value
Total Fat 1.5 g	0 %
Saturated Fat 0 g	0 %
Trans Fat 0 g	
Monounsaturated Fat 1 g	
Cholesterol 0 mg	0 %
Sodium 150 mg	7 %
Total Carbohydrates 47 g	17 %
Dietary Fiber 4 g	13 %
Sugars 12 g	
Protein 6 g	
Vitamin A 3 %	Vitamin C 3 %
Calcium 2 %	Iron 7 %
Vitamin K 30 mcg	
Potassium 200 mg	

Rice and Lentil Pilaf

Servings: 2 | Serving size: about 2 cups

Cooking time: 45 minutes

This recipe can easily be multiplied and keeps well in the refrigerator. Reheat gently.

1 quart	water
1/4 cup	black lentils
1 1/2 cups	water
1/4 cup	brown rice
1 tsp.	sesame oil
1 small	onion (diced)
1 small (4 ounce)	zucchini (cut into large dice)
1/4 tsp.	salt
to taste	fresh ground black pepper
1/2 tsp.	dried oregano

Place the water in a large stock pot over high heat.

Add the lentils and cook over a moderate boil for about 25 minutes.

Check the degree of doneness about every 3 minutes after 20 minutes and cook until just tender.

While the lentils are cooking, place the 1 1/2 cup water in a small sauce pan over high heat and bring to a boil.

Add the rice and cover. Reduce the heat until the rice is at a simmer.

Cook for about 35-40 minutes until the water has evaporated and remove from the heat. Keep covered.

While the rice and lentils are cooking place the sesame oil in a medium non-stick skillet over medium heat and add the onions.

Cook slowly until they begin to soften.

Increase the heat to medium-high and add the zucchini, salt, pepper and oregano.

Cook, tossing frequently, until the zucchini begins to brown on all sides.

Drain the cooked lentils well and add to the zucchini.

Add the cooked rice to the zucchini and lentils and stir until well blended.
Serve.

The refrigerator light goes on...
I know that this recipe uses three pans. There are recipes for pilaf that are one pot and they work OK but I have found that cooking the lentils separate from the rice and veggies keeps the flavors fresher and more distinct. The clean up is not too much problem -- all three pans wipe clean with just a bit of soap and water.

Nutrition Facts	
Serving size	about 2 cups
Servings	2
Calories 210	Calories from Fat 32
	% Daily Value
Total Fat 3.5 g	4 %
Saturated Fat 0.5 g	3 %
Trans Fat 0 g	
Monounsaturated Fat 1 g	
Cholesterol 0 mg	0 %
Sodium 300 mg	13 %
Total Carbohydrates 38 g	14 %
Dietary Fiber 5 g	17 %
Sugars 4 g	
Protein 9 g	
Vitamin A 0 %	Vitamin C 15 %
Calcium 2 %	Iron 12 %
Vitamin K 6 mcg	
Potassium 400 mg	

Dirty Rice

Servings: 2 | Serving size: 1/2 cups rice, cooked

Cooking time: 60 minutes

This recipe can easily be multiplied and makes good leftovers.

1/4 tsp.	salt
1/2 cup	brown rice
2 tsp.	olive oil
1 large	shallot (minced)
1/2 large	green bell pepper (seeded and diced)
1/2 large	red bell pepper (seeded and diced)
1/4 tsp.	ground cumin
1/2 tsp.	chili powder
1/2 tsp.	dried oregano
1/8 tsp.	cayenne (to taste)

In a medium-size saucepan, heat 2 1/2 cups water and the salt. When the liquid comes to a boil, stir in the brown rice.

Lower the heat to medium-low and simmer, covered, for 40 to 45 minutes. Do not boil away all of the liquid and do not stir the rice.

When a very small amount of liquid remains (about 1 tablespoon), remove the pan from the burner and let it stand, covered, for 3 minutes.

While the rice is cooking, heat the oil in a medium-size skillet over medium heat. Add the shallots and cook for 1 minute, stirring occasionally.

Add the peppers and cook for about 5 minutes, stirring frequently.

Add the cumin, chili powder, oregano, and cayenne.

Cook for about 1 minute, stirring until the spices are well blended.

When cooked, set the veggies aside until the rice is done.

When the rice is cooked and has stood for 3 minutes, add the spiced veggies to the rice and stir well.

Serve.

The refrigerator light goes on...
You can make rice dirty any way you like. Use whatever leftover veggies that you have. Celery, carrots, peppers, onions, mushrooms will all work well. If you want the rice less spicy, leave out the cayenne.

Nutrition Facts	
Serving size about 1 1/2 cups cooked rice	
Servings	2
Calories 240	Calories from Fat 54
	% Daily Value
Total Fat 6 g	8 %
Saturated Fat 1 g	5 %
Trans Fat 0 g	
Monounsaturated Fat 4 g	
Cholesterol 0 mg	0 %
Sodium 320 mg	14 %
Total Carbohydrates 42 g	15 %
Dietary Fiber 4 g	14 %
Sugars 4 g	
Protein 5 g	
Vitamin A 9 %	Vitamin C 96 %
Calcium 8 %	Iron 8 %
Vitamin K 10 mcg	
Potassium 300 mg	

Mashed Yams with Sage

Servings: 4 | Serving size: about one cup

Cooking time: 30 minutes

This recipe can easily be multiplied and makes good leftovers. It will keep well in the refrigerator for about 48 hours. Reheat gently.

1 cup	water
1 lb.	yams (peeled and cubed)
1 tsp.	extra virgin olive oil
1 small	shallot (minced)
1 tsp.	rubbed sage
1/8 tsp.	salt
to taste	fresh ground black pepper
2 tsp.	unsalted butter
1 Tbsp.	reduced-fat sour cream
1 Tbsp.	2% milk

Place the water in a large stock pot fitted with a steamer basket over high heat.

Add the cubed yams to the steamer basket and steam until they break slightly with a fork.

While the yams are cooking place the olive oil in a small skillet over medium heat. Add the shallots and rosemary and cook gently until the shallots are softened.

Place the cooked yams together with the shallot and rosemary mixture in a bowl. Add the salt, pepper, spread and buttermilk and mash with a fork until smooth. Add the 2% milk slowly as the yams are mashed smooth.

The mashed yams can be reheated gently in a microwave.

The refrigerator light goes on...
This is the perfect recipe to substitute for mashed potatoes. The same creamy mashed potato dish that's so comforting with the twist of added flavor. And the added benefit of more fiber!

Nutrition Facts	
Serving size	1 cup
Servings	4
Calories 210	Calories from Fat 54
	% Daily Value
Total Fat 6 g	10 %
Saturated Fat 2 g	12 %
Trans Fat 0 g	
Monounsaturated Fat 3 g	
Cholesterol 11 mg	3 %
Sodium 169 mg	6 %
Total Carbohydrates 35 g	14 %
Dietary Fiber 5 g	17 %
Sugars 1 g	
Protein 3 g	
Vitamin A 11 %	Vitamin C 34 %
Calcium 3 %	Iron 7 %
Vitamin K 10 mcg	
Potassium 1020 mg	

Zucchini with Sun Dried Tomatoes

Servings: 2 | Serving size: about 1 1/2 cups

Cooking time: 30 minutes

This recipe can easily be multiplied and leftovers are fair.

4 medium	sun dried tomato slices
1/3 cup	boiling water
1 tsp.	olive oil
1 Tbsp.	pine nuts
2 medium	zucchini (1/2 inch dice)
1/8 tsp.	salt
1/4 tsp.	dried thyme leaves
to taste	fresh ground black pepper
1 tsp.	unsalted butter

Place a large skillet over medium heat. Add the olive oil and after about a minute add the sun dried tomato and pinenuts.

Cook, stirring frequently, for about 5 minutes. Reduce the heat if necessary so that the pinenuts don't brown too much -- they should be a light golden brown.

Add the zucchini, salt, thyme and pepper. Increase the heat to medium high. Cook, tossing frequently, until the zucchini just begins to brown on all sides and is slightly soft.

The refrigerator light goes on...
This goes well with almost any dish, but especially a steak or roasted pork main course. The zucchini is simple to prep. Cut the stem end off and make three slices lengthways so you have 4 slices. Stack two slices and cut lengthways three times again. Do this with all four slices and then cut crossways for a large dice..

Nutrition Facts	
Serving size	1 1/2 cups
Servings	4
Calories 100	Calories from Fat 63
	% Daily Value
Total Fat 7 g	9 %
Saturated Fat 1.5 g	8 %
Trans Fat 0 g	
Monounsaturated Fat 3 g	
Cholesterol <5 mg	0 %
Sodium 170 mg	7 %
Total Carbohydrates 9 g	3 %
Dietary Fiber 3 g	9 %
Sugars 7 g	
Protein 4 g	
Vitamin A 1 %	Vitamin C 41 %
Calcium 3 %	Iron 8 %
Vitamin K 20 mcg	
Potassium 700 mg	

Thick Cut Yam Fries

Servings: 2 | Serving size: about 1 1/2 cups fries

Cooking time: 30 minutes

This recipe can easily be multiplied, but like most fries, does not make very good leftovers.

2 small	yams (about 5 ounces each)
2 quarts	ice water
1/4 tsp.	salt
to taste	fresh ground black pepper
1/8 tsp.	dried thyme leaves
	spray olive oil

Scrub the yams well and then cut into wedges. It's easiest to cut them in half lengthwise and then quarters and then eighths.

Place the cut yams in the ice water for 20 minutes

Place a large skillet in the oven and set the pre-heat to 325°F.

When the oven is hot spray the pan lightly with oil.

Remove the yams from the ice water and pat dry.

Add the yam wedges to the hot pan and sprinkle the salt, pepper and thyme over the top.

Spray lightly with olive oil.

Return the pan to the oven and cook for about 25 minutes tossing frequently.

Serve hot.

The refrigerator light goes on...
This recipe is so simple you just have to do it. The prep takes all of two minutes. Tossing them into a pan and watching them another 20 minutes. Great fries to go with that burger in 25-30 minutes total. Easy!

Nutrition Facts	
Serving size	about 1 1/2 cups fries
Servings	2
Calories 120	Calories from Fat 0
	% Daily Value
Total Fat 0 g	0 %
Saturated Fat 0 g	0 %
Trans Fat 0 g	
Monounsaturated Fat 0 g	
Cholesterol 0 mg	0 %
Sodium 370 mg	16 %
Total Carbohydrates 29 g	10 %
Dietary Fiber 4 g	15 %
Sugars 6 g	
Protein 2 g	
Vitamin A 112 %	Vitamin C 4 %
Calcium 3 %	Iron 5 %
Vitamin K 4 mcg	
Potassium 500 mg	

Beef Stew

Servings: 6 | Serving size: 2 1/2 cups

Cooking time: 90 minutes

I would not multiply this recipe but it can be halved. Leftovers are better than fresh.

4 cups	water
25	pearl onions (peeled)
1/3 cup	all purpose flour
1 tsp.	salt
1/4 tsp.	fresh ground black pepper
1 1/2 lbs.	flank steak (3/4 inch cubes)
	spray olive oil
1/2 lb.	button mushrooms (quartered)
1 cup	white onion (sliced)
1 Tbsp.	lemon juice
1 Tbsp.	Worcestershire sauce
1 lb.	carrots (peeled & sliced 1/4 inch thick)
2	bay leaves
1 1/2 lbs.	red potatoes (cut into 3/4 inch cubes)
1/8 tsp.	ground allspice
4 cups	water

Heat water in a medium stockpot over high heat until it is at a shiver. Add pearl onions and cook for about ten minutes. Drain and place the onions in a large stock pot.

Preheat oven to 400°F.

Mix flour, salt and pepper in a paper bag. Toss the cubes of flank steak in the flour, coating well.

Coat a large skillet with spray olive oil and heat over medium-high heat. Add cubes of flank steak and cook, turning until all sides are brown. Do not overcrowd the beef or the meat will steam and not brown. Remove the meat to the stock pot as it browns.

Add the onions to the skillet and cook until they are soft and brown. Add them to the stock pot. Add the lemon juice and Worcestershire sauce to the skillet and deglaze the pan, scraping up anything stuck to the bottom of the pan. Add the deglazing liquid to the stock pot.

Add carrots, bay leaves, potatoes, allspice, and water to the stock pot.

Place covered pot in the oven. Cook for one hour, stirring gently every fifteen minutes.

The refrigerator light goes on...
Don't stir stews too often or the potatoes will break down. Gently stir the stew, at most, about every 15 minutes.

Nutrition Facts		
Serving size		about 2 1/2 cups
Servings		8
Calories 360	Calories from Fat 81	
		% Daily Value
Total Fat 9 g		11 %
Saturated Fat 3.5 g		18 %
Trans Fat 0 g		
Monounsaturated Fat 3.5 g		
Cholesterol 75 mg		25 %
Sodium 560 mg		24 %
Total Carbohydrates 42 g		15 %
Dietary Fiber 6 g		22 %
Sugars 10 g		
Protein 30 g		
Vitamin A 70 %	Vitamin C 26 %	
Calcium 7 %	Iron 21 %	
Vitamin K 20 mcg		
Potassium 1400 mg		

Minestrone

Servings: 8 | Serving size: about 2 cups

Cooking time: 60 minutes (does not include overnight soaking of beans)

This keeps well for about 4 days in the fridge. Reheat gently. Serve with a side salad of your choice.

1 lb.	great northern beans
2 quarts	water
2 tsp.	olive oil
3 cloves	garlic (minced)
2 cups	onion (diced)
1/2 lb.	parsnips (peeled and sliced)
1/2 lb.	carrots (peeled and sliced)
3 ribs	celery (sliced)
4 cups	water
Rind (about 3" x 3")	Parmigiano-Reggiano
3	bay leaves
4 cups	non fat chicken stock
1 1/2 lbs.	red potatoes (peeled and cubed)
2 - 28 oz. cans	peeled whole tomatoes (drain & seed tomatoes)
1/2 tsp.	salt
1 Tbsp.	flat leaf parsley (per serving) (minced)
1 Tbsp.	Parmigiano-Reggiano (per serving) (grated)

Rinse beans thoroughly.

Cover beans with water and allow to soak overnight. Drain and rinse. Place in a stock pot and add two quarts water to cover.

Simmer over medium heat for 30 - 45 minutes until the beans just begin to turn soft. Drain.

While the beans are cooking heat oil in a large stock pot over medium. Add the minced garlic. Cook garlic in oil slowly. Do not allow this to brown or the garlic will become bitter. Add onion and cook slowly until it just begins to turn soft.

Add the parsnips, carrots and celery and cook over medium-low heat until the vegetables begin to soften. Cover with the water and chicken stock and add the potatoes and the rind of parmesan. Cook

over medium-low heat for about 20 minutes until the potatoes begin to soften. Add the tomatoes, beans and salt. Cook for about 20 minutes and remove the rind of parmesan.

Serve each 2 cup serving with 1 tablespoon minced parsley and grated parmesan. As with most soups, this one is best made a day in advance.

The refrigerator light goes on...
This soup, as with most soups, is best the second or third day. It is so good and so good for you making a batch in the dead of winter to have for dinner and then a few lunches will make you feel so warm. If you are out of an ingredient, that's OK. There are plenty of substitutions. Almost any root vegetable will do.

Nutrition Facts		
Serving size		2 cups
Servings		4
Calories 405	Calories from Fat 51	
		% Daily Value
Total Fat 6 g		9 %
Saturated Fat 2 g		12 %
Trans Fat 0 g		
Monounsaturated Fat 2 g		
Cholesterol 7 mg		2 %
Sodium 569 mg		24 %
Total Carbohydrates 70 g		23 %
Dietary Fiber 18 g		71 %
Sugars 12 g		
Protein 23 g		
Vitamin A 107 %	Vitamin C 71 %	
Calcium 33 %	Iron 36 %	
Vitamin K 88 mcg		
Potassium 1935 mg		

Split Pea Soup

Servings: 4 | Serving size: about 2 cups

Cooking time: 120+ minutes

This recipe can easily be multiplied and is better the next day. Store tightly covered in the refrigerator.

Serve with a 2 ounce whole grain roll and a side salad of your choice.

2 quarts	water
1 cup	split peas
1 tsp.	olive oil
2 oz.	prosciutto ham (diced)
1 large	onion (diced)
2 cups	no salt added vegetable stock
4 cups	water
1/4 tsp.	salt
to taste	fresh ground black pepper
1/4 tsp	ground nutmeg
2 Tbsp.	dry sherry

Place the split peas in the boiling water and cook at a rolling boil for 2 minutes and remove from heat.

Let stand for an hour and drain.

Place the olive oil in a 4 quart sauce pan over medium heat.

Add the diced ham and cook slowly for five minutes until the ham is not quite crispy.

Add the onion and increase the heat slightly.

Cook, stirring frequently, until the onions begin to be soft.

Add the split peas and stir well.

Add the vegetable stock, water and salt and cook for about an hour over low-medium heat. Stir occasionally.

When the split peas are slightly soft, remove the pan from the heat.

Remove about 1 1/2 cups of the soup and puree the remaining using a stick blender or blender.

Add the 1 1/2 cups of split peas back to the soup and stir.

Add the nutmeg and sherry and cook for another 5 minutes.

Serve.

The refrigerator light goes on...
I loved split pea soup as a kid and this is the flavor that I crave every now and then.

Back then I think it was the economical choice - a bit of ham, split peas, onion - a super simple dish that pairs perfectly with a sandwich or salad. The thing is that people don't think of it as an upscale choice, but a bit of nutmeg and sherry really elevates the soup.

Serve this with an egg salad sandwich or a grilled cheese sandwich and you have a wonderful meal for a cold night.

Nutrition Facts	
Serving size	2 cups
Servings	4
Calories 240	Calories from Fat 27
	% Daily Value
Total Fat 3 g	5 %
Saturated Fat 0.5 g	3 %
Trans Fat 0 g	
Monounsaturated Fat 1.5 g	
Cholesterol 10 mg	3 %
Sodium 340 mg	15 %
Total Carbohydrates 36 g	13 %
Dietary Fiber 13 g	47 %
Sugars 7 g	
Protein 15 g	
Vitamin A 0 %	Vitamin C 4 %
Calcium 2 %	Iron 14 %
Vitamin K 8 mcg	
Potassium 500 mg	

Creamy Chicken and Potato Soup

Servings: 4 | Serving size: about 2 cups

Cooking time: 60 minutes

This recipe can easily be multiplied by 2. As with almost all soups this recipe is better the next day.

2 tsp.	olive oil
1 large	red onion (diced)
2 large	carrots (peeled and diced)
1 clove	garlic (minced)
2 cups	no salt added chicken stock
1/2 cup	water
1/4 tsp.	salt
1 lb.	Yukon gold potatoes (cut into 1 inch cubes)
to taste	fresh ground black pepper
1 lb.	boneless chicken breast (cut into 1/2 inch cubes)
1 cup	2% milk
3 Tbsp.	fresh dill

Place the olive oil in a large stock pot over medium heat. Add the red onion and cook for about 3 minutes.

Add the carrots and garlic and cook for another 5 minutes until the onions begin to turn translucent.

Add the chicken stock, water, salt, and potatoes. Season with pepper and reduce the heat to low.

Simmer for about 50 minutes. Stir occasionally. Cook until the potatoes are soft and beginning to fall apart.

Add the chicken breast and fresh dill. Stir and then slowly add the milk. Cook for another ten minutes.

Serve.

The refrigerator light goes on...
This is a quick and easy soup. It does take a bit of time to simmer -- just long enough to watch Jeopardy -- but it's perfect on a cold night -- warm, creamy and really filling. All of that with 5 grams of fiber and tons of vitamins.

Nutrition Facts	
Serving size	2 cups
Servings	4
Calories 310	Calories from Fat 63
	% Daily Value
Total Fat 7 g	9 %
Saturated Fat 2 g	9 %
Trans Fat 0 g	
Monounsaturated Fat 2.5 g	
Cholesterol 85 mg	28 %
Sodium 270 mg	12 %
Total Carbohydrates 32 g	12 %
Dietary Fiber 5 g	19 %
Sugars 10 g	
Protein 31 g	
Vitamin A 35 %	Vitamin C 21 %
Calcium 4 %	Iron 8 %
Vitamin K 8 mcg	
Potassium 1200 mg	

Lentil Soup

Servings: 4 | Serving size: about 2 cups.

Cooking time: 60 minutes

This recipe can easily be multiplied, and like many soups, this recipe is better the second day.

1 Tbsp.	olive oil
1 large	white onion (diced)
2 ribs	celery (diced)
2 large	carrots (peeled and diced)
4 ounces	sliced ham (cut into small dice)
1/2 tsp.	salt
to taste	fresh ground black pepper
1 cup	dried lentils
1 Tbsp.	dried sage (crumbled)
2	bay leaves
1/2 tsp.	dried thyme leaves
2 cups	no salt added chicken stock
8 cups	water

Place the olive oil in a large sauce pan over medium heat. Add the onion and cook for about 5 minutes and add the celery and carrots.

Cook, stirring frequently, for about 5 minutes and add the ham.

Cook, stirring frequently, for about 5 minutes and add the salt, pepper, lentils, sage, bay leaves, thyme chicken stock and water.

Stir well and reduce the heat to medium-low Cook for about 45 minutes until the lentils are soft.

The refrigerator light goes on...
This is the perfect soup for autumn. Pair this with a simple side salad and you have the best fall meal going. I look for ham that's as low in sodium as I can find. The Healthy Choice is a pretty good pick but there are a lot of sliced hams on the market that are minimally processed with no nitrates and are much lower in sodium.

Nutrition Facts	
Serving size	2 cups
Servings	4
Calories 300	Calories from Fat 63
	% Daily Value
Total Fat 7 g	8 %
Saturated Fat 1.5 g	7 %
Trans Fat 0 g	
Monounsaturated Fat 3.5 g	
Cholesterol 15 mg	5 %
Sodium 710 mg	31 %
Total Carbohydrates 44 g	16 %
Dietary Fiber 8 g	30 %
Sugars 7 g	
Protein 19 g	
Vitamin A 34 %	Vitamin C 13 %
Calcium 6 %	Iron 22 %
Vitamin K 30 mcg	
Potassium 700 mg	

Vitamin K Content of Foods

Short list

This is the down and dirty list-one that you can keep on hand so that you know what foods to avoid.

High (over 40 mcg Vitamin K per serving)

Vegetables	Serving Size	mcg per serving
Spinach, frozen	10 oz.	1189.5
Parsley, raw	1 cup	984.0
Spinach, cooked	1 cup	888.5
Collard Greens, cooked	1 cup	836.0
Kale, raw, chopped	1 cup	547.4
Swiss Chard, raw	1 cup	298.8
Mustard greens, raw, chopped	1 cup	278.5
Broccoli, cooked, chopped	1 cup	220.2
Brussels sprouts, cooked	1 cup	218.8
Onions, green/scallions, raw	1 cup	207.0
Brussels sprouts, raw	1 cup	155.8
Spinach, raw	1 cup	144.9
Turnip greens, raw	1 cup	138.1
Endive, raw, chopped	1 cup	115.6
Broccoli, raw, chopped	1 cup	92.5
Watercress, raw	1 cup	85.0
Okra, cooked	1 cup	64.0
Lettuce, green leaf, raw	1 cup	62.5
Peas, green, frozen, cooked	10 oz	60.7
Lettuce, Boston/Bibb, raw	1 cup	56.3
Leek, raw	1 medium	41 8
Lettuce, Romaine, raw	1 cup	48.2
Cabbage, napa, raw, shredded	1 cup	42.0
Peas, green, cooked	1 cup	41.4
Peas, sugar snap, cooked	1 cup	40.0

Legumes and Beans		mcg per serving
Soybeans (edamame)	1 cup	87.4

Misc.		mcg per serving
Cilantro, fresh	9 sprigs	62.0

Medium (between 20 and 40 mcg Vitamin K per serving)

Vegetables	Serving Size	mcg per serving
Lettuce, red leaf, raw	1 cup	39.3
Asparagus, cooked	5 spears	38.0
Spaghetti/Marinara sauce	1 cup	34.8
Asparagus, raw	5 spears	33.5
Cabbage, red, raw, shredded	1 cup	26.7
Lettuce, Iceberg, raw	2 cups	26.6
Cabbage, Chinese, raw, shredded	1 cup	25.1
Tomatoes, sun-dried	1 Cup	23.2
Peas & onions, frozen, cooked	1 cup	21.8
Carrots, cooked, slices	1 cup	21.4
Cauliflower, cooked	1 cup	21.4

Fruits	Serving Size	mcg per serving
Pumpkin, canned	1 cup	39.2
Kiwi fruit	1 medium	30.6
Blackberries	1 cup	28.5
Blueberries	1 cup	28.0
Grapes, red/green, seedless	1 cup	23.4

Legumes and Beans	Serving Size	mcg per serving
Bean sprouts, mung, fresh	1 cup	34.3
Cashews	½ cup	23.8

Misc.	Serving Size	mcg per serving
Thyme, dried	1 tsp	24.0

Comprehensive list

This is nearly a complete list of the foods used in this book that you can use for reference if you have a question about a particular ingredient.

Vegetables	Serving Size	mcg per serving
Anchovies, fillets	1 each	0.5
Asparagus, raw	5 spears	33.5
Asparagus, cooked	5 spears	38.0
Beans, green, cooked	1 cup	20.0
Beans, yellow (wax beans), raw	1 cup	0.0
Beets, cooked, sliced	1 cup	0.40
Broccoli, raw, chopped	1 cup	92.5
Broccoli, cooked, chopped	1 cup	220.2
Brussels sprouts, cooked	1 cup	218.8
Brussels sprouts, raw	1 cup	155.8
Cabbage, Chinese, raw, shredded	1 cup	25.1
Cabbage, napa, raw, shredded	1 cup	42.0
Cabbage, red, raw, shredded	1 cup	26.7
Carrots, raw, strips or slices	1 cup	16.1
Carrots, cooked, slices	1 cup	21.4
Cauliflower, raw	1 cup	16.0
Cauliflower, cooked	1 cup	21.4
Celery	1 stalk	11.7
Collard Greens, cooked	1 cup	836.0
Corn, yellow, cooked	1 cup	0.7
Corn, yellow, raw	1 cup	0.5
Cucumber	1 medium	14.5
Eggplant, raw, cubed	1 cup	2.9
Eggplant, cooked, cubed	1 cup	2.9
Endive, raw, chopped	1 cup	115.6
Fennel	1 bulb	0
Garlic	3 cloves	0.1
Kale, raw, chopped	1 cup	547.4
Leek, raw	1 medium	41
8Lettuce, arugula	1/2 cup	10.9
Lettuce, Boston/Bibb, raw	1 cup	56.3
Lettuce, green leaf, raw	1 cup	62.5
Lettuce, red leaf, raw	1 cup	39.3
Lettuce, Romaine, raw	1 cup	48.2
Lettuce, Iceberg, raw	1 cup	13.3
Mushrooms, raw	1 cup	0
Mustard greens, raw, chopped	1 cup	278.5
Okra, cooked	1 cup	64.0
Onions, green/scallions, raw	1 cup	207.0
Onions, white/red/yellow, raw	1 cup	0.6
Parsley, raw	1 cup	984.0

Parsnips, cooked	1 cup	1.6
Peas, green, frozen, cooked	10 oz	60.7
Peas, green, cooked	1 cup	41.4
Peas & onions, frozen, cooked	1 cup	21.8
Peas, sugar snap, cooked	1 cup	40.0
Pepper, green bell	1 medium	8.8
Pepper, jalapeno	1 medium	1.4
Pepper, red bell	1 medium	5.8
Pepper, red chili, hot	1 each	6.3
Pepper, yellow sweet	1medium	0
Potato, red, cooked	1 medium	4.8
Potato, white, baked	1 medium	4.7
Potato, sweet, cooked	1 medium	2.6
Shallots, chopped	1 Tbsp	0
Snow peas, raw	1 cup	15.8
Spaghetti/Marinara sauce	1 cup	34.8
Spinach, raw	1 cup	144.9
Spinach, cooked	1 cup	888.5
Spinach, frozen	10 oz.	1189.5
Squash, acorn	1 cup	0
Squash, butternut, cooked, cubed	1 cup	2.0
Squash, summer, cooked	1 cup	6.3
Swiss Chard, raw	1 cup	298.8
Tomato paste	1 Tbsp	1.8
Tomato, plum	1	4.9
Tomato, raw	1 medium	9.7
Tomato sauce, canned, no salt	1 cup	6.8
Tomatoes, canned, whole	1 cup	7.7
Tomatoes, cherry	1 cup	11.8
Tomatoes, sun-dried	1 Cup	23.2
Turnips, cooked	1 cup	0.2
Turnip greens, raw	1 cup	138.1
Watercress, raw	1 cup	85.0]
Zucchini, cooked	1 cup	7.6

Fruits

Apple, with peel	1 medium	3.0
Apple, peeled	1 medium	0.8
Applesauce	1 cup	1.5
Avocado	1/4	10.5
Banana	1 medium	0.6
Blackberries	1 cup	28.5
Blueberries	1 cup	28.0
Cantaloupe, cubed	1 cup	4.0
Cherries, no pits	1 cup	3.0
Cranberries, dried	1/3 cup	1.5

Cranberries, raw	1/3 cup	1.9
Currants	1/2 cup	0
Grapes, red/green, seedless	1 cup	23.4
Kiwi fruit	1 medium	30.6
Lemon	1 medium	0
Lime	1 medium	0
Mango	1 cup	6.9
Melon, cantaloupe, diced	1 cup	3.9
Melon, honeydew, diced	1 cup	4.9
Orange	1 medium	0
Orange peel	1 tsp.	0
Peach	1 medium	2.5
Pear	1 medium	7.5
Pineapple, fresh, diced	1 cup	1.1
Plum	1 each	4.2
Prunes, dried	2 each	10.0
Pumpkin, canned	1 cup	39.2
Raisins	½ cup	2.5
Strawberries, fresh, sliced	1 cup	3.2
Watermelon, fresh, cubed	1 cup	0.2

Meats

Bacon, pork, cooked	2 strips	0
Beef, cooked, lean	3.5 ounces	1.5
Beef, ground, fried, lean	3.5 ounces	1.4
Beef stock	1 cup	0.2
Chicken, cooked, breast, no skin	3.5 ounces	0.3
Chicken stock	1 cup	0.5
Clams, canned, chopped	1 can	0.3
Clams, fresh	3.5 ounces	0
Crabmeat, cooked	1 cup	0.1
Fish, cod, cooked	3.5 ounces	0.1
Fish, grouper, cooked	3.5 ounces	0
Fish, haddock, cooked	3.5 ounces	0
Fish, halibut, cooked	3.5 ounces	0
Fish, salmon, cooked	3.5 ounces	0
Fish, sole, cooked	3.5 ounces	0.1
Fish, tuna, cooked	3.5 ounces	0
Fish, tuna, canned	3.5 ounces	2.5
Lamb, cooked	3.5 ounces	0
Liver, beef, cooked	3.5 ounces	3.3
Mussels, cooked	3.5 ounces	0
Pork, cooked	3.5 ounces	0
Scallops, cooked	3.5 ounces	0.2
Shrimp, cooked	3.5 ounces	0
Turkey, cooked, no skin	3.5 ounces	0

Turkey pepperoni	3.5 ounces	0
Turkey sausage, cooked	3.5 ounces	1.5

Starches

Bagel	1 whole	0
Biscuit	1	0
Bread, white/wheat/rye	1 slice	0.8
Bulgar, cooked	1 cup	0.9
Cornbread	1 piece – 2.5 x 2.5-inch	0
Cornmeal, blue	100 grams	0
Cornmeal, yellow	1 cup	0.4
Cornstarch	1 cup	0
Couscous, cooked	1 cup	0.2
Crackers, saltine	4 squares	0
Crackers, graham	2 squares	0.8
Croutons, plain	1 cup	0
English muffin	1	0
Flour	1cup	0.4
Grits, cooked	1 cup	0
Melba toast, plain	1 cup, rounds	0.3
Pasta, dry	1 oz	0
Rice, white & brown, cooked	1 cup	0
Rice, wild, cooked	1 cup	0.8
Tortilla, corn, 6-inch	1 each	0
Tortilla, flour, 6-inch	1 each	1.0

Cereals

Barley, dry	1/4 cup	1.0
Cereal, oatmeal	1 cup	1.2
Cereal, cream of wheat	1 cup	0.3
Grits, cooked	1 cup	0

Legumes and Beans

Almonds	1 oz	0
Bean sprouts, mungo, fresh	1 cup	34.3
Beans, black, dried, cooked	1 cup	0
Beans, garbanzo, canned	1 cup	0
Beans, great northern, dried, cooked	1 cup	0
Beans, great northern, canned	1 cup	0
Beans, kidney, dried, cooked	1 cup	14.9
Beans, kidney, canned	1 cup	5.6
Beans, red kidney, dried, cooked	1 cup	5.8
Beans, red kidney, canned	1 cup	10.5
Beans, lima, dried, cooked	1 cup	3.8
Beans, navy, dried, cooked	1 cup	1.1
Beans, navy, canned	1 cup	7.6
Beans, pinto, dried, cooked	1 cup	6.0
Beans, pinto, canned	1 cup	5.3
Cashews	1/2 cup	23.8
Lentils, dry, cooked	1/4 cup	3.4
Peanuts	2 Tbsp	0
Peanut butter, low fat	1/4 cup	0
Pecans, chopped	1 cup	3.8
Pine nuts	1 oz	15.3
Pistachio nuts	1 cup	0
Soybeans (ddamame)	1 cup	87.4
Tahini	1 Tbsp	0
Tofu	3.5 oz	0
Walnuts, chopped	1 cup	3.2

Dairy

Buttermilk, non-fat	1 cup	0.2
Cheese, blue	1 oz	0.7
Cheese, cheddar	1 oz	0.8
Cheese, cheddar, reduced fat	1 oz	0.2
Cheese, cottage	1 cup	0.9
Cheese, feta	1 oz	0.5
Cheese, fontina	1 oz	0.7

Cheese, goat	1 oz	0.7
Cheese, monteray	1 oz	0.7
Cheese, mozzarella, part skim	1 oz	0.4
Cheese, parmesan	1 oz	0.5
Cheese, ricotta, reduced fat	1 cup	1.7
Cheese, swiss, low fat	1 oz	1.7
Egg, whole, large	1 each	0.1
Egg, white, large	1 each	0
Egg, yolk large	1 each	0.1
Egg substitute	1 cup	2.0
Milk, 2 percent	1 cup	0.2
Milk, dry, non-fat	1 cup	0.1
Milk, coconut	1 cup	0
Milk, evaporated, non-fat	1 cup	0
Milk, dry, non fat	1 cup	0.1
Milk, soy	1 cup	7.3
Milk, whole	1 cup	0.5
Sour cream, non fat	1 cup	0
Yogurt, plain, low-fat	1 cup	0.5

Beverages

Beer	12 oz	0
Bourbon	1 oz	0
Carbonated soda	12 oz	0
Coffee, brewed	1 cup	0.2
Coffee, instant, granules	1 tsp	0
Grapefruit juice	1 cup	0
Lemon juice	1 oz	0
Lime juice	1 oz	0.2
Orange juice	1 cup	0.2
Sake	1 oz	0
Tea, brewed	1 cup	0
Tomato juice, canned, no salt	1 cup	5.6
V-8 juice	1 cup	12.8
Vodka	1 oz	0
Wine	1 cup	0

Fats

Butter	1 tsp.	0.3
Cream cheese	1 Tbsp.	0.4

Mayonnaise, reduced calorie	1 Tbsp.	3.6
Oil, canola	1 tsp.	5.5
Oil, corn	1 tsp.	0.1
Oil, grapeseed	1 tsp.	0
Oil, olive	1 tsp.	2.7
Oil, peanut	1 tsp.	0
Oil, safflower	1 tsp.	0.3
Oil, sesame	1 tsp.	0.6
Oil, soybean	1 tsp.	8.9
Sour cream	1 Tbsp.	0.1

Misc.

Allspice	1 tsp	0
Baking powder	1 tsp	0
Baking soda	1 tsp	0
Basil, fresh	5 leaves	10.4
Bay leaves, crushed	1 tsp	0
Capers	1 Tbsp	2.1
Cardamom, ground	1 tsp	0
Celery Seed	1 tsp	0
Chili powder	1 tsp	2.7
Chives	1 Tbsp	6.4
Cilantro, fresh	9 sprigs	62.0
Cinnamon, ground	1 tsp	0.7
Cloves, ground	1 tsp	3.0
Cumin, seed	1 tsp	0.1
Curry powder	1 tsp	2.0
Dill, fresh	5 sprigs	0
Garlic powder	1 tsp	0
Gelatin, dry, unflavored	1 envelope	0
Ginger, ground	1 tsp	0
Ginger root	1 tsp	0
Ketchup	1 Tbsp	0.3
Marjoram, ground	1 tsp	3.7
Mint	2 Tbsp	0
Mustard	1 Tbsp	0.4
Mustard, seed	1 tsp	0.2
Nutmeg, ground	1 tsp	0
Olives, ripe, canned	3.5 oz	1.4
Oregano, dried	1 tsp	6.2
Paprika	1 tsp	1.7
Pepper	1 tsp	3.4
Pepper, red, ground	1 tsp	1.4
Pickle, dill	1 medium	11.9
Pickle, gherkin	1 medium	19.1

Relish	1 Tbsp	2.5
Rosemary	1 tsp	0
Saffron	1 Tbsp	0
Sage, ground	1 tsp	12.0
Salt	1 tsp	0
Sesame seeds	1 tsp	0
Soy sauce	1 Tbsp	0
Tarragon, dried	1 tsp	0
Tabasco sauce	1 tsp	0
Thyme, dried	1 tsp	24.0
Vanilla extract	1 tsp	0
Vinegar	1 Cup	0
Wasabi root	1	0
Worcestershire sauce	1 Tbsp	0.2
Yeast, dry, active	1 tsp	0

Sweets

Chocolate, bakers, bittersweet	1 square	2.8
Chocolate syrup	2 Tbsp	0.1
Cocoa, dry, powered	2 Tbsp	0
Gelatin, fruit flavored	1 cup	0
Graham crackers	2-1/2 square	0.3
Maple syrup	1 Tbsp	0
Pie, apple	1 piece	4.4
Pudding	1 cup	0
Sherbet	1 cup	0
Splenda	1 tsp	0
Sugar, white or brown	1 Tbsp.	0
Honey	1 Tbsp.	0
Jam/jelly	1 Tbsp.	0
Jam/jelly, apricot	1 Tbsp	0.1
Wafer, chocolate	1 each	0.1

Made in the USA
Middletown, DE
04 November 2023

41830844R00077